Low-Fodmap Diet Cookbook

A New Beginning with Deliciously Simple Recipes for Digestive Bliss & IBS Management. Includes 60-Days Meal Plan

Cotry Jordan

Table Of Content

Chapter 1: Introduction to the Low-Fodmap Journey

Embarking on the journey of understanding and managing IBS (irritable bowel syndrome) and various digestive disorders is a significant step towards reclaiming control over one's health and well-being. This introduction delves into the complex world of digestive health, illuminating the intricacies of IBS, and unravelling the science behind the Low-Fodmap diet, a proven approach to alleviate and manage these conditions. We will also share inspiring success stories, offering a glimpse into the transformative power of this diet on individuals' lives.

Understanding IBS and Digestive Disorders

IBS, a common disorder affecting the large intestine, presents a spectrum of symptoms including abdominal pain, bloating, gas, diarrhea, and constipation. Its exact causes remain elusive, often making diagnosis and treatment a challenging process. The complexity of IBS lies in its variability; it's a condition deeply influenced by an individual's diet, lifestyle, and stress levels. In addition to IBS, other digestive disorders such as Crohn's disease, ulcerative colitis, and celiac disease, although distinct in their pathology, share commonalities in how they impact the gut and overall quality of life.

The journey to understanding these conditions begins with recognizing their multifaceted nature. They are not just disorders of the gut but are conditions that can profoundly affect mental health, personal relationships, and day-to-day functioning. To manage them effectively, a holistic approach is required, one that encompasses medical intervention, dietary adjustments, and lifestyle changes.

The Science Behind the Low-Fodmap Diet

Enter the Low-Fodmap diet, a scientifically-backed dietary plan developed by researchers at Monash University. FODMAPs, an acronym for Fermentable Oligosaccharides, Disaccharides, Monosaccharides, and Polyols, are short-chain carbohydrates that are poorly absorbed in the small intestine.

When these carbohydrates ferment in the gut, they can trigger symptoms in individuals with a sensitive digestive system.

The Low-Fodmap diet involves a three-phase approach: elimination, reintroduction, and personalization. In the elimination phase, high-Fodmap foods are removed from the diet for a period, usually 4-6 weeks. This phase often brings significant relief for many, highlighting the impact of these foods on their symptoms. The reintroduction phase involves systematically adding high-Fodmap foods back into the diet to identify specific triggers. Finally, the personalization phase is about creating a long-term, sustainable diet that avoids individual triggers but remains nutritionally balanced.

This diet is not a one-size-fits-all solution but a personalized journey to understand one's body and its reactions to different foods. It empowers individuals to make informed choices about their diet, leading to a better quality of life.

Success Stories: Transformations and Testimonials

The transformative impact of the Low-Fodmap diet is best illustrated through the stories of those who have walked this path. These are tales of individuals who, burdened by the debilitating effects of digestive disorders, found relief and a new lease on life through this dietary change. Their journeys are marked by challenges, learning, and ultimately, triumph.

These stories are not just about the alleviation of physical symptoms but about regaining confidence, joy, and freedom in life. They speak of restored social interactions, where dining out is no longer a source of anxiety but a pleasure. They talk about renewed energy levels, enabling individuals to pursue hobbies and activities they once loved but had to give up due to their condition.

Above all, these testimonials stand as a beacon of hope for anyone starting their Low-Fodmap journey. They reinforce the idea that while the path might be challenging, the destination – a life of fewer symptoms and greater enjoyment – is within reach.

In summary, this introductory chapter sets the stage for a deeper exploration into the world of IBS and digestive disorders, the science behind the Low-Fodmap diet, and the real-life stories of transformation it has enabled. It is an invitation to embark on a journey of discovery, learning, and healing, guided by science, enriched by personal experiences, and aimed at achieving long-term health and happiness. As we delve into the subsequent sections, we aim to equip you with the knowledge, tools, and inspiration needed to navigate this journey successfully.

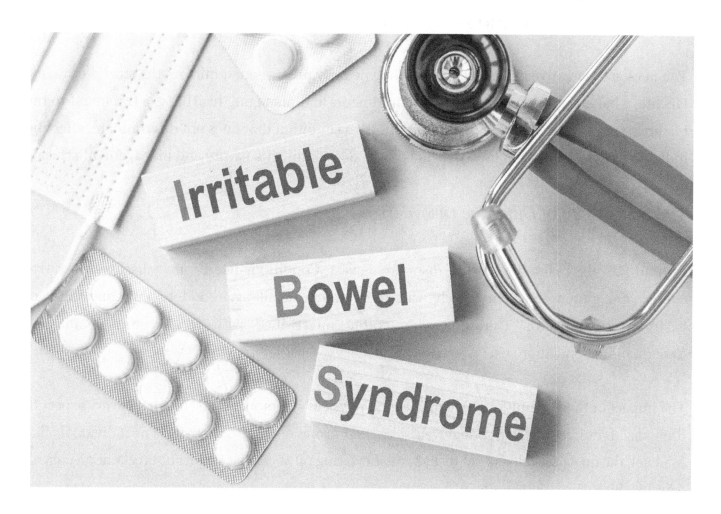

1.1. Understanding IBS and Digestive Disorders

In the heart of the bustling city, amidst the hustle of everyday life, lies an invisible battle many individuals face - the struggle with IBS and digestive disorders. This section delves into the intricacies of these conditions, shedding light on their impact and the transformative potential of the Low-Fodmap diet in managing them.

The Silent Struggle: Life with IBS

For countless individuals, irritable bowel syndrome (IBS) is a daily reality. It's a condition characterized by a symphony of symptoms - abdominal pain, bloating, constipation, and diarrhea, to name a few. The unpredictability of IBS can turn a regular day into a relentless challenge. Imagine planning your day around the proximity to restrooms, or the anxiety of dining out, not knowing if the meal will trigger your symptoms.

The personal narrative of Michael, our archetype busy professional, mirrors the stories of many. His life, a balancing act between work commitments and managing his IBS, is a testament to the resilience required to navigate this condition. It's a condition that does not discriminate, affecting individuals across ages and lifestyles, making understanding its nature and management crucial.

The Complexity of Digestive Disorders

Beyond IBS, the realm of digestive disorders is vast. Conditions like Crohn's disease, ulcerative colitis, and gluten sensitivity, each with their unique challenges, add to the complexity of gastrointestinal health. These disorders, often intertwined with IBS, require a nuanced understanding and approach.

The impact of these conditions extends beyond physical symptoms. They touch on every aspect of life - social interactions, emotional wellbeing, and professional productivity. For individuals like Michael, the quest for relief is not just about alleviating physical discomfort but reclaiming control over his life.

Transforming Lives with the Low-Fodmap Diet

Enter the Low-Fodmap diet, a scientifically-backed approach that offers a beacon of hope. This diet revolves around the reduction of certain carbohydrates that are poorly absorbed in the small intestine, known as FODMAPs. These culprits are often responsible for the uncomfortable symptoms associated with IBS and other digestive disorders.

The journey through the Low-Fodmap diet is not a one-size-fits-all solution; it's a personalized path to digestive bliss. It's about understanding your body's unique responses and crafting a diet that caters to your specific needs. For individuals like Michael, this diet is not just about dietary changes; it's a lifestyle transformation.

Through real-life examples and practical guidance, this section aims to empower individuals to take charge of their digestive health. It's about breaking down the complexities of IBS and digestive disorders, providing clarity and hope. The Low-Fodmap diet is more than a list of foods to avoid; it's a roadmap to a life of comfort and confidence.

As we embark on this journey, remember, you're not alone in this fight. The path to digestive health is a journey of discovery, resilience, and ultimately, transformation. The Low-Fodmap diet is your ally in this quest, a tool to unlock a life free from the constraints of IBS and digestive disorders.

In the following chapters, we will explore the science behind the Low-Fodmap diet, real-life success stories, and practical steps to embark on your Low-Fodmap journey. Together, we will navigate the path to digestive health and wellness, transforming challenges into triumphs.

1.2 The Science Behind the Low-Fodmap Diet

The Low-Fodmap Diet, a term that echoes with promise and potential, stands as a beacon of hope for those grappling with digestive disorders. This journey into the scientific realm of the diet is not just about understanding its principles; it's about unraveling the mysteries of our digestive system and how we can harmoniously coexist with it.

Unveiling the Mysteries of FODMAPs

FODMAPs - an acronym for Fermentable Oligosaccharides, Disaccharides, Monosaccharides, and Polyols - are a group of carbohydrates that are not easily absorbed in the small intestine. When these unabsorbed carbohydrates travel to the large intestine, they become a feast for the resident bacteria, resulting in fermentation.

This fermentation process is a natural part of digestion but, for some individuals, it can lead to symptoms like bloating, gas, stomach pain, constipation, and diarrhea.

The concept of FODMAPs was pioneered by researchers at Monash University in Australia. Their groundbreaking work demonstrated that a diet low in FODMAPs could significantly alleviate the symptoms of IBS and other functional gastrointestinal disorders. This discovery was not just a scientific breakthrough; it was a paradigm shift in how we approach dietary management of digestive health.

The Gut Microbiome: A Delicate Ecosystem

At the heart of the Low-Fodmap Diet is an understanding of the gut microbiome - the complex community of microorganisms living in our digestive system. This ecosystem plays a crucial role in our overall health, influencing digestion, immunity, and even mental wellbeing. FODMAPs, by their nature, impact this microbiome, leading to the symptoms experienced by those with sensitive guts.

The diet's approach is not about eliminating these microorganisms; rather, it's about creating an environment in the gut that favors balance and harmony. By reducing the intake of high-FODMAP foods, we decrease the fermentation that can cause distress, thereby fostering a more comfortable digestive process.

Implementing the Low-Fodmap Diet: A Scientific Approach

The implementation of the Low-Fodmap Diet is a journey of discovery and adjustment. It begins with a phase of elimination, where high-FODMAP foods are removed from the diet. This phase is crucial, as it sets the stage for identifying which foods trigger symptoms.
Following this, the reintroduction phase begins, where foods are gradually added back to the diet to pinpoint the specific FODMAPs that cause discomfort.

This methodical approach is backed by science and has proven effective in numerous studies. However, it's important to note that the diet is highly individualized. What may be a trigger for one person may not be for another. This customization is key in making the Low-Fodmap Diet a sustainable lifestyle change rather than a temporary fix.

In conclusion, the science behind the Low-Fodmap Diet is a testament to the power of dietary intervention in managing digestive disorders. It's a diet that goes beyond mere food choices; it's a lifestyle that embraces the complexity of our bodies and seeks to live in harmony with them. As we continue our journey through this book, we will explore how to prepare for your Low-Fodmap adventure, integrating this science-backed approach into your daily life for lasting digestive wellness.

1.3 Success Stories: Transformations and Testimonials

The Low-Fodmap Diet is more than a set of dietary guidelines; it's a catalyst for transformation. This chapter is dedicated to the voices of those who have journeyed through the challenges of digestive disorders and found solace and success through the Low-Fodmap Diet. Their stories are not just narratives of change; they are testaments to the resilience of the human spirit and the power of personalized nutrition.

Reclaiming Life: Personal Triumphs

At the core of each success story is an individual who faced the daily struggles of a digestive disorder. These are not just tales of dietary changes but of life reclaimed. For instance, consider the story of John, a 45-year-old engineer, whose life was once dictated by the unpredictable bouts of IBS.

John's journey began with skepticism but led to a remarkable transformation. By adhering to the Low-Fodmap Diet, he not only alleviated his symptoms but also discovered a newfound passion for cooking and nutrition.

Then there's Emma, a 38-year-old graphic designer and mother of two, who battled with chronic bloating and discomfort. Emma's story is one of perseverance and discovery. The Low-Fodmap Diet not only eased her physical symptoms but also brought a sense of control and creativity to her meals. These personal triumphs extend beyond the realm of health; they touch on the essence of living a fuller, more vibrant life.

Beyond Symptom Relief: Holistic Wellness

The impact of the Low-Fodmap Diet goes beyond symptom relief; it often sparks a journey towards holistic wellness. Individuals find themselves more attuned to their bodies, developing a deeper understanding of how food influences their overall well-being. This newfound awareness transcends dietary choices, influencing lifestyle changes that encompass exercise, mindfulness, and mental health.

Take, for example, the experience of Alex, a 40-year-old entrepreneur. His adherence to the Low-Fodmap Diet not only mitigated his IBS symptoms but also led him to embrace a more active lifestyle and mindfulness practices. This holistic approach resulted in improved energy levels, better stress management, and an overall enhanced quality of life.

Community Voices: Collective Wisdom

The power of community cannot be understated in the journey of dietary transformation. The testimonials and experiences shared by individuals who have embraced the Low-Fodmap Diet create a tapestry of collective wisdom.
This wisdom is not just in the successful management of symptoms but in the shared tips, recipes, and encouragement that form a supportive network.

Online forums, social media groups, and local meetups have become hubs for sharing experiences and advice. Here, newcomers to the diet find inspiration and guidance, while seasoned adherents offer insights and support. This communal aspect of the Low-Fodmap journey fosters a sense of belonging and solidarity, proving that no one has to navigate this path alone.

The success stories and testimonials present in this chapter are more than individual achievements; they are a chorus of voices that echo the efficacy and life-changing potential of the Low-Fodmap Diet. They serve as beacons of hope and sources of inspiration for anyone embarking on this journey. As we delve into the following chapters, these stories will act as a backdrop, reminding us of the real-life impact and transformative power of this dietary approach.

As we conclude this opening chapter, it's essential to reflect on the key themes and insights that have emerged in our exploration of IBS and digestive disorders, the science of the Low-Fodmap diet, and the powerful testimonials of those who have found relief and transformation through this dietary journey. This conclusion aims to weave these strands together, offering a comprehensive overview and inspiring guidance for those embarking on their Low-Fodmap journey.

Holistic Understanding of Digestive Health

The journey into the world of IBS and digestive disorders has underscored the importance of a holistic understanding of health. We have seen how these conditions are not just physical ailments but encompass a range of psychological, social, and emotional dimensions. The interplay between diet, stress, and gut health forms a complex web where each element impacts the other. This understanding is crucial for anyone dealing with these conditions, as it highlights the need for a comprehensive approach to management and treatment.

Empowerment through Knowledge and Science

The exploration of the Low-Fodmap diet has provided a scientific foundation to approach IBS and other related digestive disorders. Understanding the role of FODMAPs in triggering symptoms empowers individuals to make informed dietary choices. The diet's phased approach – elimination, reintroduction, and personalization – offers a structured path to identify specific triggers and develop a customized diet that suits one's unique needs.

This empowerment through knowledge is a critical aspect of the journey. It transforms patients from passive sufferers to active participants in their health management. It equips them with the tools to take control of their symptoms and, by extension, their lives.

Inspirational Stories of Transformation

Perhaps the most compelling aspect of this chapter has been the success stories. These narratives have brought to life the transformative potential of the Low-Fodmap diet. They have shown us that while the journey may be challenging, it is also replete with opportunities for growth, learning, and ultimately, healing.

These stories are a testament to the resilience of the human spirit and the body's ability to heal when given the right conditions. They remind us that change is possible, that relief from symptoms is achievable, and that a better quality of life can be attained.

A Journey of Continuous Learning and Adaptation

As we move forward from this introductory chapter, it's important to remember that the Low-Fodmap journey is one of continuous learning and adaptation. What works for one person may not work for another, and what works at one point in time may need to be adjusted as circumstances change.

This journey requires patience, persistence, and a willingness to experiment and learn from both successes and setbacks. It involves staying updated with the latest research, consulting with healthcare professionals, and perhaps most importantly, listening to one's own body and its responses to different foods.

A Call to Action: Embracing the Journey

As we conclude, this chapter serves as a call to action for anyone struggling with IBS or related digestive disorders. The journey to managing these conditions through the Low-Fodmap diet is a path worth exploring. It offers hope and a concrete way to not just manage symptoms but to improve overall quality of life.

We encourage readers to approach this journey with an open mind, a spirit of inquiry, and a commitment to self-care. It's a journey that may challenge you, but it also holds the promise of profound personal transformation and relief.

In closing, the Low-Fodmap journey is more than a dietary change; it's a pathway to a new understanding of your body, your health, and your well-being. It's an opportunity to live a fuller, more vibrant life, free from the constraints of digestive discomfort. As you turn the page to the next chapter, remember that this journey is not just about the destination but about the insights, growth, and discoveries you make along the way.

Chapter 2: Preparing for Your Low-Fodmap Adventure

As you embark on the transformative Low-Fodmap journey, Chapter 2 serves as your practical guide to seamlessly integrating this new dietary approach into your daily life. Transitioning to a Low-Fodmap diet requires more than just a list of foods to avoid; it involves a holistic reorientation of your kitchen habits, shopping strategies, and understanding of essential ingredients. This introduction lays out the foundational steps to effectively prepare for your Low-Fodmap adventure, ensuring you are well-equipped to manage your digestive health with confidence and ease.

Transforming Your Kitchen into a Low-Fodmap Haven

The first step in your Low-Fodmap adventure is reimagining your kitchen space. This transformation is not merely about removing high-Fodmap foods; it's about creating an environment that supports your new dietary needs. Setting up your Low-Fodmap kitchen involves a thoughtful reorganization of pantry staples, cooking utensils, and storage solutions. This process also includes understanding cross-contamination and how to prevent it, especially in households where not everyone is following the same diet.

A Low-Fodmap kitchen is more than a physical space; it's a mindset shift towards mindful and health-conscious cooking. This includes embracing new cooking techniques that preserve the nutritional integrity of Low-Fodmap ingredients and experimenting with alternative methods to recreate favorite dishes within the diet's guidelines.

Mastering the Art of Smart Shopping

Navigating grocery stores on a Low-Fodmap diet can be daunting at first. With a plethora of food choices, deciphering what aligns with your dietary needs is key.
This section will provide you with strategies to shop smartly, from reading and understanding food labels to identifying hidden Fodmaps in packaged foods.

We'll explore how to plan your grocery trips effectively, making them less overwhelming and more productive. You'll learn how to stock your pantry with Low-Fodmap essentials, ensuring you always have the right ingredients on hand to whip up a gut-friendly meal. This part of the journey is not just about avoiding certain foods; it's about discovering a variety of new, wholesome, and delicious options.

Essential Low-Fodmap Ingredients and Substitutes

One of the most exciting aspects of embarking on a Low-Fodmap diet is the exploration of new ingredients and substitutes. This section of the chapter will introduce you to a range of essential Low-Fodmap ingredients that will become the building blocks of your meals. Understanding these ingredients' roles and how they can be used creatively in cooking will open up a world of culinary possibilities.

We will delve into the art of substitution, showing you how to replace high-Fodmap ingredients with Low-Fodmap alternatives without compromising on taste or texture. This knowledge is crucial in maintaining the variety and enjoyment in your diet, making the Low-Fodmap lifestyle not just manageable but enjoyable.

A Journey of Learning and Adaptation

As you progress through this chapter, remember that adapting to a Low-Fodmap diet is a journey of learning and adaptation. It's about developing new habits, gaining new knowledge, and continually adjusting your approach as you discover what works best for you. This chapter aims to equip you with the tools and knowledge you need to make this transition as smooth and stress-free as possible.

In conclusion, preparing for your Low-Fodmap adventure is an integral part of managing your digestive health. This chapter will guide you through setting up your Low-Fodmap kitchen, shopping smart, and understanding essential Low-Fodmap ingredients and substitutes. By the end of this chapter, you will have a solid foundation to confidently embark on your Low-Fodmap journey, empowered by the knowledge that you have the tools and resources to make it a success.

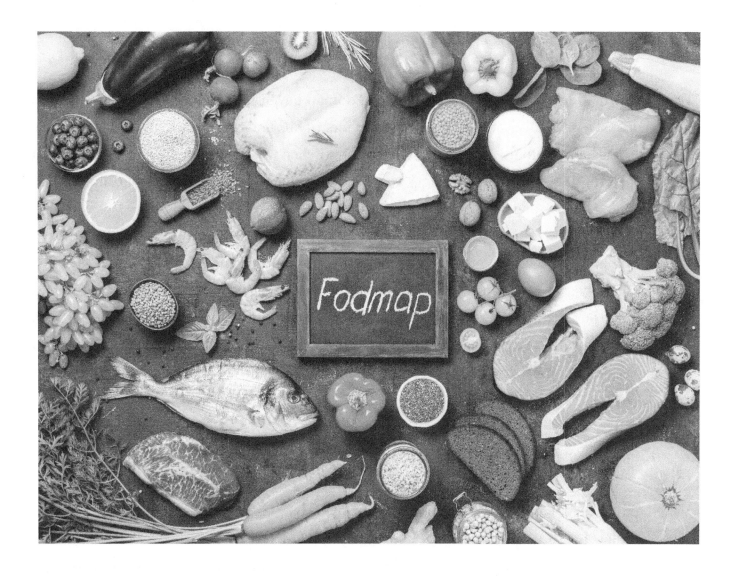

2.1. Setting Up Your Low-Fodmap Kitchen

Embarking on the Low-Fodmap diet is akin to setting sail on a voyage of culinary discovery. This journey, while exciting, requires preparation and the right tools. Setting up your kitchen is the first step in making this diet a seamless part of your daily routine. It's not just about removing certain foods; it's about creating a space that supports your dietary needs and inspires your culinary creativity.

Creating a Low-Fodmap Friendly Environment

The transformation of your kitchen into a Low-Fodmap haven begins with decluttering. This is more than just a physical cleaning; it's a process of identifying and removing high-FODMAP foods that could trigger symptoms. This doesn't mean your kitchen will be bare or your meals bland. On the contrary, this is an opportunity to stock your shelves with an array of Low-Fodmap alternatives that are both delicious and nourishing.

Start by familiarizing yourself with high-FODMAP ingredients commonly found in kitchens. Items like garlic, onions, wheat-based products, certain dairy products, and various fruits and vegetables might need to be substituted. Replace these with Low-Fodmap alternatives like garlic-infused oils, gluten-free grains, lactose-free dairy, and a rainbow of suitable fruits and vegetables. This swap not only ensures compliance with the diet but also introduces a variety of new flavors and textures to explore.

Equipping Your Kitchen for Success

A well-equipped kitchen is a cornerstone of successful meal preparation, especially when following a specific diet. Invest in quality kitchen tools that make the preparation of Low-Fodmap meals both easy and enjoyable. A good set of knives, cutting boards, pots, and pans are essential. Additionally, consider gadgets like a slow cooker or a food processor, which can be incredibly handy for preparing Low-Fodmap meals efficiently.

Organizing your kitchen plays a crucial role in simplifying your cooking experience. Group your Low-Fodmap ingredients together, perhaps in a specific cabinet or section of your pantry. This not only saves time but also reduces the risk of accidentally using high-FODMAP ingredients. Labeling shelves and containers can be a helpful way to ensure that everything you need for your Low-Fodmap meals is readily at hand.

Stocking Up on Low-Fodmap Staples

A key aspect of setting up your Low-Fodmap kitchen is stocking it with the right ingredients. Building a pantry filled with Low-Fodmap staples ensures that you always have the necessary components for a quick, delicious, and compliant meal. This includes items like gluten-free flours, quinoa, rice, oats, lactose-free dairy products, and Low-Fodmap nuts and seeds.

Herbs and spices are your allies in adding flavor to your meals without adding FODMAPs. Fresh herbs like basil, chives, and coriander, as well as an array of dried spices, can transform your dishes. Additionally, consider having a collection of Low-Fodmap condiments and sauces to add quick flavor to any meal.

Setting up your Low-Fodmap kitchen is an integral part of your journey towards better digestive health. It's about creating a space that not only complies with your dietary needs but also inspires and facilitates the joy of cooking. A well-prepared kitchen is the foundation upon which delicious, nutritious, and symptom-free meals are built. As you continue through this book, you will find numerous recipes and ideas to fill your Low-Fodmap kitchen with delectable dishes, making each meal a step towards digestive wellness and culinary delight.

2.2. Shopping Smart: Navigating Grocery Stores

Mastering the art of grocery shopping is a pivotal skill in your Low-Fodmap adventure. The aisles of a grocery store are like a maze, filled with options that can either support or derail your dietary goals. This chapter is dedicated to transforming you into a savvy shopper, someone who can navigate the complexities of food labels and make choices that align with your Low-Fodmap needs.

Strategic Planning: The Key to Smart Shopping

The foundation of smart grocery shopping is strategic planning. Before stepping into the store, arm yourself with a well-thought-out shopping list. This list should be based on the meal plans you intend to follow, taking into consideration the portion sizes and frequency of meals. By having a clear list, you can avoid impulse buys that may not be Low-Fodmap friendly.

Additionally, familiarize yourself with the layout of the grocery store you frequent. Most stores are designed with fresh produce, dairy, and meat sections along the perimeter. These areas typically house the most Low-Fodmap friendly options. The inner aisles, while they do contain necessary items like gluten-free grains and canned goods, can also be laden with high-FODMAP temptations. Navigating the store with an understanding of its layout can save time and reduce the risk of falling off the Low-Fodmap wagon.

Deciphering Food Labels: Your Roadmap to Safe Choices

In the world of Low-Fodmap eating, understanding food labels is crucial. Labels are your roadmap to identifying ingredients that are safe and those that should be avoided. Look for key high-FODMAP ingredients like onion, garlic, high-fructose corn syrup, and wheat. If any of these are present, it's a signal to steer clear of that product.

However, it's not just about avoiding high-FODMAP foods; it's also about finding nutritious alternatives. For instance, instead of wheat-based pasta, look for varieties made from rice, quinoa, or corn. When selecting dairy products, opt for lactose-free versions or plant-based alternatives like almond or coconut milk.

Building a Low-Fodmap Pantry: Essential Purchases

Building a Low-Fodmap pantry is an ongoing process. Each shopping trip is an opportunity to gradually stock your pantry with staples that form the backbone of your Low-Fodmap diet. Essentials like gluten-free grains, rice, oats, quinoa, and a variety of nuts and seeds are versatile and can be used in multiple recipes. Canned goods like chickpeas, lentils, and tomatoes (without added high-FODMAP ingredients) are also handy for quick and nutritious meals.

Spices and herbs are invaluable in adding flavor to your meals without adding FODMAPs. Stock up on Low-Fodmap friendly options like ginger, basil, thyme, and oregano. Remember, fresh herbs typically have lower FODMAP levels compared to their dried counterparts.

Becoming a smart shopper is an essential part of your Low-Fodmap journey. It's about being prepared, understanding labels, and making informed choices that support your dietary needs. With each grocery trip, you'll gain more confidence in selecting foods that contribute to your digestive wellness and culinary satisfaction. This chapter is your guide to mastering the grocery aisles, ensuring that your Low-Fodmap kitchen is always well-stocked with the right ingredients.

2.3. Essential Low-Fodmap Ingredients and Substitutes

Mastering the art of grocery shopping is a pivotal skill in your Low-Fodmap adventure. The aisles of a grocery store are like a maze, filled with options that can either support or derail your dietary goals. This chapter is dedicated to transforming you into a savvy shopper, someone who can navigate the complexities of food labels and make choices that align with your Low-Fodmap needs.

Strategic Planning: The Key to Smart Shopping

The foundation of smart grocery shopping is strategic planning. Before stepping into the store, arm yourself with a well-thought-out shopping list. This list should be based on the meal plans you intend to follow, taking into consideration the portion sizes and frequency of meals. By having a clear list, you can avoid impulse buys that may not be Low-Fodmap friendly.

Additionally, familiarize yourself with the layout of the grocery store you frequent. Most stores are designed with fresh produce, dairy, and meat sections along the perimeter. These areas typically house the most Low-Fodmap friendly options. The inner aisles, while they do contain necessary items like gluten-free grains and canned goods, can also be laden with high-FODMAP temptations. Navigating the store with an understanding of its layout can save time and reduce the risk of falling off the Low-Fodmap wagon.

Deciphering Food Labels: Your Roadmap to Safe Choices

In the world of Low-Fodmap eating, understanding food labels is crucial. Labels are your roadmap to identifying ingredients that are safe and those that should be avoided.

Look for key high-FODMAP ingredients like onion, garlic, high-fructose corn syrup, and wheat. If any of these are present, it's a signal to steer clear of that product.

However, it's not just about avoiding high-FODMAP foods; it's also about finding nutritious alternatives. For instance, instead of wheat-based pasta, look for varieties made from rice, quinoa, or corn. When selecting dairy products, opt for lactose-free versions or plant-based alternatives like almond or coconut milk.

Building a Low-Fodmap Pantry: Essential Purchases

Building a Low-Fodmap pantry is an ongoing process. Each shopping trip is an opportunity to gradually stock your pantry with staples that form the backbone of your Low-Fodmap diet. Essentials like gluten-free grains, rice, oats, quinoa, and a variety of nuts and seeds are versatile and can be used in multiple recipes. Canned goods like chickpeas, lentils, and tomatoes (without added high-FODMAP ingredients) are also handy for quick and nutritious meals.

Spices and herbs are invaluable in adding flavor to your meals without adding FODMAPs. Stock up on Low-Fodmap friendly options like ginger, basil, thyme, and oregano. Remember, fresh herbs typically have lower FODMAP levels compared to their dried counterparts.

Becoming a smart shopper is an essential part of your Low-Fodmap journey. It's about being prepared, understanding labels, and making informed choices that support your dietary needs. With each grocery trip, you'll gain more confidence in selecting foods that contribute to your digestive wellness and culinary satisfaction. This chapter is your guide to mastering the grocery aisles, ensuring that your Low-Fodmap kitchen is always well-stocked with the right ingredients.

As we reach the conclusion of Chapter 2, "Preparing for Your Low-Fodmap Adventure," we've journeyed through the practical aspects of transitioning to a Low-Fodmap diet. From setting up your kitchen to smart grocery shopping and understanding essential ingredients and substitutes, this chapter has provided a comprehensive roadmap to help you navigate this new dietary landscape with confidence and ease. Let's consolidate the key takeaways and insights to ensure a smooth and successful continuation of your Low-Fodmap journey.

Creating a Supportive Low-Fodmap Kitchen Environment

The transformation of your kitchen into a Low-Fodmap friendly space is pivotal. It's not just about removing high-Fodmap items but creating an environment that supports your health goals. This involves organizing your pantry and fridge, understanding food storage, and minimizing cross-contamination risks. The kitchen is where your commitment to the Low-Fodmap diet materializes into action. It becomes a place where healthful and delicious meals are prepared, where the challenges of managing digestive disorders are met with proactive and positive solutions.

Empowering Yourself through Smart Shopping

Grocery shopping, often seen as a mundane task, becomes an empowering activity on your Low-Fodmap journey. Learning to read labels carefully, understanding the nuances of Fodmap content, and making informed choices about what to put in your cart is empowering. It's about gaining control over your diet and, by extension, your symptoms. The ability to navigate grocery aisles with confidence is a significant step towards independence and assurance in managing your dietary needs.

Discovering the Versatility of Low-Fodmap Ingredients

One of the most enlightening aspects of this chapter has been the exploration of essential Low-Fodmap ingredients and their substitutes. This part of your journey is characterized by discovery and creativity. It opens up a new world of flavors and textures, showing that a diet designed to ease digestive discomfort doesn't have to be bland or restrictive. Learning to substitute high-Fodmap ingredients with Low-Fodmap alternatives broadens your culinary repertoire and ensures that your diet remains diverse and enjoyable.

The Journey Ahead: Continuous Learning and Adaptation

As we wrap up this chapter, it's important to remember that the transition to a Low-Fodmap diet is a continuous process of learning and adaptation. It's normal to face challenges along the way – whether it's a mistakenly consumed high-Fodmap food or the initial complexity of label reading.

What's important is the commitment to stay on course, learn from these experiences, and continually adapt your approach.

The journey ahead is not just about adhering to a list of do's and don'ts. It's about listening to your body, understanding its responses, and adjusting accordingly. It's about developing a deeper connection with food and how it affects your health. This journey is as much about nourishing your body as it is about fostering resilience, patience, and self-awareness.

Conclusion: Embarking on Your Low-Fodmap Adventure with Confidence

As you embark on your Low-Fodmap adventure, equipped with the knowledge and tools from this chapter, do so with confidence and optimism. You have taken the first crucial steps in managing your digestive health and improving your quality of life. The path ahead is not just a culinary adjustment but a journey towards wellness and discovery.

Remember, the Low-Fodmap diet is a personal journey. What works for one person may not work for another. Stay flexible, be open to experimenting, and most importantly, be kind to yourself as you navigate this new way of eating. You are not just changing your diet; you are taking control of your health and well-being.

In closing, let this chapter serve as a foundation upon which you build your Low-Fodmap lifestyle. As you move forward, carry the lessons, insights, and skills you have acquired. Know that each step you take is a step towards better health and a more vibrant life. The journey may have its challenges, but the rewards – a life with less discomfort and more enjoyment – are well worth the effort.

Chapter 3: The Low-Fodmap Lifestyle

3.1. Balancing Nutrition on a Low-Fodmap Diet

The Low-Fodmap Diet, primarily designed to ease digestive discomfort, can sometimes inadvertently lead to nutritional imbalances if not carefully managed. This chapter is dedicated to guiding you through the process of maintaining a nutritionally balanced diet while adhering to Low-Fodmap guidelines. It's about ensuring that your body receives all the nutrients it needs to thrive, even when certain food groups are limited or eliminated.

Understanding Nutritional Needs on a Low-Fodmap Diet

The key to balancing nutrition on a Low-Fodmap diet is understanding the nutritional profile of the foods you can eat and how they contribute to your overall dietary needs. The diet restricts certain fruits, vegetables, grains, and dairy products – all of which are common sources of essential nutrients like vitamins, minerals, and fiber.

- *Protein:* Protein is crucial for muscle repair, immune function, and overall health. Ensure adequate protein intake by including Low-Fodmap options like lean meats, fish, eggs, and certain plant-based proteins like tempeh.
- *Carbohydrates:* While many high-Fodmap foods are carbohydrate-rich, there are plenty of Low-Fodmap grains and starches like rice, potatoes, and quinoa that provide the necessary energy and fiber.
- *Fats:* Healthy fats are essential for hormone production and cell health. Include sources like olive oil, nuts (like walnuts and peanuts), and seeds (like chia and pumpkin seeds) in your diet.
- *Vitamins and Minerals:* A varied intake of Low-Fodmap fruits and vegetables, along with fortified foods or supplements as necessary, can help maintain adequate vitamin and mineral levels.

Strategic Meal Planning: Ensuring a Balanced Diet

Strategic meal planning is pivotal in achieving a balanced diet on Low-Fodmap regimen. It involves more than just avoiding triggers; it's about creating meals that are rich in nutrients, variety, and flavor.

- **Diverse Food Selection:** Aim for diversity in your meals to ensure a broad spectrum of nutrients. Incorporate different colors of fruits and vegetables, a variety of protein sources, and an array of grains and healthy fats.
- **Portion Control:** Pay attention to portion sizes, especially when it comes to Low-Fodmap foods that have a threshold for tolerance. Eating moderate amounts can help avoid inadvertently triggering symptoms.
- **Regular Meal Times:** Eating at regular intervals can help maintain steady energy levels and prevent overeating, which can sometimes trigger IBS symptoms.

Overcoming Nutritional Challenges: Tips and Tricks

While following a Low-Fodmap diet, certain nutritional challenges might arise. Here are some tips and tricks to tackle these challenges:

- **Fiber Intake:** With the restriction of some high-fiber foods, maintaining adequate fiber intake can be challenging. Include Low-Fodmap sources of fiber like oats, quinoa, carrots, and oranges to help meet your daily fiber needs.
- **Calcium and Vitamin D:** With the limitation on certain dairy products, ensure adequate calcium and vitamin D intake through fortified non-dairy milks, leafy greens, and supplements if necessary.
- **Iron Absorption:** For those relying on plant-based iron sources, combine them with vitamin C-rich foods to enhance absorption. For example, pair spinach with bell peppers or tofu with a squeeze of lemon juice.

Balancing nutrition on a Low-Fodmap diet requires mindful planning and an understanding of the nutritional value of Low-Fodmap foods. By focusing on a diverse and balanced intake, portion control, and strategic nutrient pairing, you can ensure that your diet is not only effective in managing IBS symptoms but also supportive of your overall health and well-being. This chapter serves as a guide to help you navigate the nutritional aspects of the Low-Fodmap diet, making it a sustainable and healthful lifestyle choice.

3.2. Mindful Eating and Digestive Health

In the journey of managing digestive health, particularly within the framework of the Low-Fodmap diet, the concept of mindful eating emerges as a powerful tool. This chapter delves into the practice of mindful eating and its profound impact on digestive health. It's not merely about the foods you eat; it's about how you eat them, your relationship with food, and the awareness you bring to each meal.

The Essence of Mindful Eating

Mindful eating is the practice of being fully present and engaged with the eating experience. It involves paying attention to the flavors, textures, and sensations of your food, as well as your body's hunger and fullness cues. This practice stands in stark contrast to the mindless eating habits common in today's fast-paced lifestyle, where meals are often consumed quickly, in front of screens, or on-the-go.

- *Engaging the Senses:* Start by appreciating the appearance and aroma of your food. As you eat, try to identify all the flavors and textures. This sensory engagement can enhance your enjoyment of the meal and lead to a deeper appreciation for the foods that nourish your body.
- *Listening to Your Body:* Mindful eating also involves tuning into your body's signals. Eat slowly and pay attention to how your body feels. Are you still hungry, or are you beginning to feel full? Learning to recognize these cues can prevent overeating, which is often a trigger for digestive discomfort.

Mindful Eating and the Low-Fodmap Diet

Adhering to the Low-Fodmap diet requires a heightened awareness of what you eat. Mindful eating complements this by adding an awareness of how you eat. This combination can be particularly beneficial in managing IBS and other digestive disorders.

- **Identifying Triggers:** By eating mindfully, you may be able to better identify foods that trigger symptoms. This awareness can be crucial in customizing the Low-Fodmap diet to suit your individual needs.
- **Reducing Stress Eating:** Stress can exacerbate digestive symptoms. Mindful eating encourages a more relaxed and focused approach to meals, which can help in managing stress-related digestive issues.
-

Practical Tips for Integrating Mindful Eating into Your Lifestyle

Incorporating mindful eating into your daily routine doesn't have to be daunting. Here are some practical tips to get started:

- **Create a Calm Eating Environment:** Reduce distractions during meals. Turn off the TV and put away your phone. Try to eat at a table rather than on the couch or at your desk.
- **Slow Down:** Chew your food thoroughly and put down your utensils between bites. This not only aids digestion but also gives your body time to recognize satiety.
- **Reflect on Your Food Choices:** Consider the nutritional value and Low-Fodmap compliance of your food. This reflection can help you make choices that are both satisfying and supportive of your digestive health.
- **Practice Gratitude:** Take a moment before each meal to express gratitude. This can shift your mindset and enhance your overall eating experience.
-

Mindful eating is more than a practice; it's a lifestyle change that can significantly improve your relationship with food and its impact on your digestive health. By embracing the principles of mindful eating, you can enhance the effectiveness of the Low-Fodmap diet, manage symptoms more effectively, and cultivate a more harmonious relationship with food. This chapter serves as a guide to help you integrate mindful eating into your Low-Fodmap lifestyle, paving the way for improved digestive health and overall well-being.

3.3. Incorporating Exercise and Wellness

In the comprehensive approach to managing IBS and following the Low-Fodmap diet, exercise and overall wellness play crucial roles. This chapter is not just about the physical act of exercising; it's about integrating physical activity into your lifestyle in a way that supports your digestive health and overall well-being. Here, we explore the symbiotic relationship between exercise, wellness, and the Low-Fodmap diet.

The Impact of Exercise on Digestive Health

Exercise is a powerful ally in the management of IBS and digestive discomfort. Regular physical activity has been shown to improve bowel movements, reduce stress (a known trigger for IBS symptoms), and enhance overall digestive function.

- **Stress Reduction:** Activities like yoga, tai chi, and moderate walking can significantly reduce stress levels, which in turn can alleviate IBS symptoms.
- **Improving Gut Motility:** Regular exercise, especially cardiovascular activities like jogging, swimming, or cycling, can help in enhancing gut motility and regularity.

Tailoring Exercise to Your Low-Fodmap Lifestyle

While exercise is beneficial, it's important to tailor it to fit your Low-Fodmap lifestyle and current health status. Here's how you can integrate exercise into your routine:

- **Listen to Your Body:** Pay attention to how your body responds to different types of exercises. Some people may find high-intensity workouts trigger their symptoms, while others may thrive on them.
- **Hydration and Nutrition:** Ensure proper hydration and fuel your body with Low-Fodmap snacks or meals before and after workouts. This will help maintain energy levels and prevent any exercise-induced digestive issues.
- **Consistency Over Intensity:** Aim for regular, moderate exercise rather than sporadic, intense workouts. Consistency helps in building a routine that your body can adapt to more easily.

Holistic Wellness: Beyond Exercise

Wellness extends beyond physical exercise; it encompasses mental and emotional health, which are deeply intertwined with digestive health.

- ***Mindfulness and Relaxation Techniques:*** Practices like meditation, deep breathing, and progressive muscle relaxation can help in managing the psychological aspects of IBS.
- ***Sleep Hygiene:*** Adequate and quality sleep is vital. Poor sleep can exacerbate digestive issues, so focus on establishing a regular sleep schedule and creating a restful sleeping environment.
- ***Social Connections and Support:*** Building a supportive community, whether it's through IBS support groups, exercise classes, or social activities, can provide emotional support and reduce feelings of isolation often associated with chronic health issues.
-

Integrating Wellness into Everyday Life

To effectively integrate wellness into your life, consider the following:

- ***Create a Balanced Routine:*** Balance your day with periods of activity and relaxation. Incorporate short walks during breaks and relaxation techniques in the evening.
- ***Be Flexible and Forgiving:*** Some days might be harder than others. Be flexible with your routine and forgiving of yourself on days when your symptoms might flare up.
- ***Celebrate Small Wins:*** Acknowledge and celebrate the small victories, whether it's sticking to your exercise routine, trying a new relaxation technique, or successfully managing your symptoms for a day.

Exercise and overall wellness are integral components of managing IBS and optimizing your health on the Low-Fodmap diet. By finding the right balance and types of exercise, incorporating relaxation and mindfulness practices, and focusing on holistic wellness, you can create a lifestyle that supports both your digestive and overall health. This chapter provides the tools and insights to help you build a well-rounded approach to wellness, tailored to your unique needs and lifestyle.

Chapter 4: Energizing Breakfasts

4.1. Quick and Easy Morning Starters

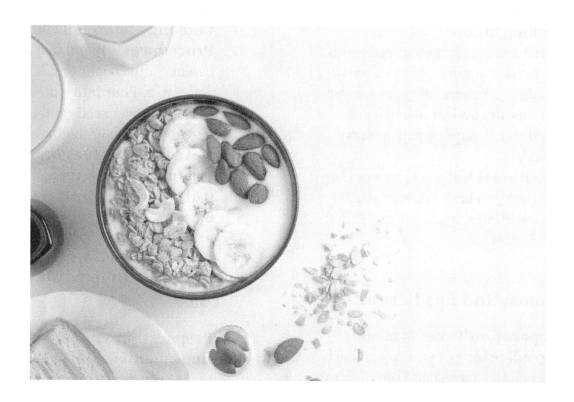

Banana Almond Oatmeal

- **Preparation Time:** 10 minutes
- **Ingredients:** 1 cup rolled oats, 2 cups almond milk, 1 ripe banana (mashed), 1 teaspoon cinnamon, 1 tablespoon almond butter
- **Servings:** 2
- **Cooking Method:** Simmering

- **Procedure:** 1. Combine oats and almond milk in a saucepan. 2. Simmer on low heat until oats are soft. 3. Stir in mashed banana, cinnamon, and almond butter. 4. Cook for another 2 minutes. 5. Serve warm.
- **Nutritional Values (per serving):** Calories: 285 kcal, Protein: 8g, Carbohydrates: 49g, Fat: 7g, Fiber: 6g, Sugars: 12g

Chia Seed Yogurt Parfait

- **Preparation Time:** 15 minutes
- **Ingredients:** 1/2 cup chia seeds, 1 cup lactose-free yogurt, 1 cup strawberries (sliced), 1 tablespoon maple syrup
- **Servings:** 2
- **Cooking Method:** Layering
- **Procedure:** 1. Mix chia seeds with lactose-free yogurt. 2. Let sit for 10 minutes. 3. In serving glasses, layer chia mixture and strawberries. 4. Drizzle with maple syrup. 5. Serve chilled.
- **Nutritional Values (per serving):** Calories: 320 kcal, Protein: 10g, Carbohydrates: 45g, Fat: 12g, Fiber: 15g, Sugars: 18g

Spinach and Egg Scramble

- **Preparation Time:** 15 minutes
- **Ingredients:** 3 eggs, 1 cup spinach (chopped), 1 tablespoon olive oil, salt and pepper to taste
- **Servings:** 2
- **Cooking Method:** Scrambling
- **Procedure:** 1. Beat eggs with salt and pepper. 2. Heat olive oil in a skillet. 3. Add spinach, cook until wilted. 4. Pour in eggs, scramble until cooked. 5. Serve hot.
- **Nutritional Values (per serving):** Calories: 200 kcal, Protein: 14g, Carbohydrates: 2g, Fat: 15g, Fiber: 1g, Sugars: 1g

Raspberry Smoothie Bowl

- **Preparation Time:** 10 minutes
- **Ingredients:** 1 cup frozen raspberries, 1 banana, 1/2 cup coconut milk, 1 tablespoon sunflower seeds, 1 teaspoon honey
- **Servings:** 1
- **Cooking Method:** Blending
- **Procedure:** 1. Blend raspberries, banana, and coconut milk until smooth. 2. Pour into a bowl. 3. Top with sunflower seeds and a drizzle of honey. 4. Serve immediately.
- **Nutritional Values (per serving):** Calories: 280 kcal, Protein: 4g, Carbohydrates: 40g, Fat: 12g, Fiber: 8g, Sugars: 22g

Feta and Olive Gluten-Free Toast

- **Preparation Time:** 10 minutes
- **Ingredients:** 2 slices gluten-free bread, 1/4 cup feta cheese (crumbled), 1 tablespoon black olives (chopped), 1 teaspoon olive oil
- **Servings:** 1
- **Cooking Method:** Toasting
- **Procedure:** 1. Toast gluten-free bread to desired crispness. 2. Top with crumbled feta and olives. 3. Drizzle with olive oil. 4. Serve immediately.
- **Nutritional Values (per serving):** Calories: 250 kcal, Protein: 7g, Carbohydrates: 28g, Fat: 12g, Fiber: 2g, Sugars: 4g

Peanut Butter and Banana Rice Cakes

- **Preparation Time:** 5 minutes
- **Ingredients:** 2 rice cakes, 2 tablespoons peanut butter, 1 banana (sliced), 1 teaspoon chia seeds
- **Servings:** 1
- **Cooking Method:** Assembling
- **Procedure:** 1. Spread peanut butter evenly on rice cakes. 2. Top with banana slices. 3. Sprinkle with chia seeds. 4. Serve immediately.
- **Nutritional Values (per serving):** Calories: 320 kcal, Protein: 8g, Carbohydrates: 45g, Fat: 14g, Fiber: 5g, Sugars: 18g

4.2. Comforting Warm Breakfasts

Maple Cinnamon Oat Porridge

- **Preparation Time:** 15 minutes
- **Ingredients:** 1 cup rolled oats, 2 cups almond milk, 1 tablespoon maple syrup, 1/2 teaspoon ground cinnamon, pinch of salt
- **Servings:** 2
- **Cooking Method:** Simmering
- **Procedure:** 1. Combine oats, almond milk, cinnamon, and salt in a saucepan. 2. Simmer over medium heat for 10 minutes, stirring occasionally. 3. Stir in maple syrup. 4. Serve warm.
- **Nutritional Values (per serving):** Calories: 230 kcal, Protein: 5g, Carbohydrates: 38g, Fat: 6g, Fiber: 5g, Sugars: 10g

Fluffy Scrambled Eggs with Spinach

- **Preparation Time:** 10 minutes
- **Ingredients:** 4 eggs, 1/2 cup chopped spinach, 2 tablespoons lactose-free cream, 1 tablespoon olive oil, salt and pepper to taste
- **Servings:** 2
- **Cooking Method:** Scrambling
- **Procedure:** 1. Whisk eggs, lactose-free cream, salt, and pepper. 2. Heat olive oil in a skillet. 3. Add spinach, cook until wilted. 4. Pour in egg mixture, scramble gently until set. 5. Serve hot.
- **Nutritional Values (per serving):** Calories: 270 kcal, Protein: 14g, Carbohydrates: 2g, Fat: 23g, Fiber: 1g, Sugars: 1g

Warm Quinoa and Berry Bowl

- **Preparation Time:** 20 minutes
- **Ingredients:** 1 cup cooked quinoa, 1/2 cup mixed berries (strawberries, blueberries), 1 tablespoon chia seeds, 1/2 cup almond milk, 1 teaspoon honey
- **Servings:** 1
- **Cooking Method:** Mixing
- **Procedure:** 1. Warm cooked quinoa in a bowl. 2. Top with berries and chia seeds. 3. Pour warm almond milk over the mix. 4. Drizzle with honey. 5. Serve immediately.
- **Nutritional Values (per serving):** Calories: 320 kcal, Protein: 9g, Carbohydrates: 45g, Fat: 12g, Fiber: 8g, Sugars: 10g

Savory Breakfast Rice Bowl

- **Preparation Time:** 20 minutes
- **Ingredients:** 1 cup cooked brown rice, 1/4 cup diced bell peppers, 1/4 cup diced zucchini, 1 tablespoon olive oil, 2 eggs, salt and pepper to taste
- **Servings:** 2
- **Cooking Method:** Sautéing
- **Procedure:** 1. Heat olive oil in a pan. 2. Sauté bell peppers and zucchini until tender. 3. Add cooked rice, mix well. 4. Make two wells in the rice, crack eggs into them. 5. Cover and cook until eggs are set. 6. Season with salt and pepper. 7. Serve hot.
- **Nutritional Values (per serving):** Calories: 350 kcal, Protein: 12g, Carbohydrates: 45g, Fat: 15g, Fiber: 4g, Sugars: 3g

Low-Fodmap Breakfast Hash

- **Preparation Time:** 30 minutes
- **Ingredients:** 2 medium potatoes (diced), 1/2 cup diced carrots, 1/2 cup diced pumpkin, 1 tablespoon garlic-infused oil, salt and pepper to taste, fresh parsley for garnish
- **Servings:** 2
- **Cooking Method:** Roasting
- **Procedure:** 1. Preheat oven to 200°C (400°F). 2. Toss potatoes, carrots, and pumpkin in garlic-infused oil, salt, and pepper. 3. Spread on baking sheet, roast for 25 minutes, stirring halfway. 4. Garnish with parsley. 5. Serve hot.
- **Nutritional Values (per serving):** Calories: 220 kcal, Protein: 4g, Carbohydrates: 40g, Fat: 5g, Fiber: 6g, Sugars: 5g

Lactose-Free Yogurt with Nut Granola

- **Preparation Time:** 15 minutes (plus chilling)
- **Ingredients:** 1 cup lactose-free yogurt, 1/2 cup low-Fodmap granola (nut-based), 1 tablespoon maple syrup, 1/4 cup diced kiwi
- **Servings:** 1
- **Cooking Method:** Layering
- **Procedure:** 1. In a serving bowl, layer lactose-free yogurt and low-Fodmap granola. 2. Top with diced kiwi. 3. Drizzle with maple syrup. 4. Chill for 10 minutes before serving.
- **Nutritional Values (per serving):** Calories: 310 kcal, Protein: 12g, Carbohydrates: 45g, Fat: 10g, Fiber: 4g, Sugars: 20g

4.3. On-the-Go Breakfast Ideas

Berry Banana Yogurt Smoothie

- **Preparation Time:** 5 minutes
- **Ingredients:** 1 cup lactose-free yogurt, 1/2 banana, 1/2 cup mixed berries (frozen), 1 tablespoon almond butter, 1 teaspoon honey
- **Servings:** 1
- **Cooking Method:** Blending
- **Procedure:** 1. Combine all ingredients in a blender. 2. Blend until smooth. 3. Pour into a travel cup for an on-the-go breakfast.
- **Nutritional Values (per serving):** Calories: 280 kcal, Protein: 10g, Carbohydrates: 35g, Fat: 12g, Fiber: 4g, Sugars: 20g

Gluten-Free Ham and Cheese Muffins

- **Preparation Time:** 25 minutes
- **Ingredients:** 1 cup gluten-free flour, 1/2 cup diced ham, 1/2 cup grated cheddar cheese, 2 eggs, 1/2 cup lactose-free milk, 2 tablespoons olive oil, 1 teaspoon baking powder
- **Servings:** 4
- **Cooking Method:** Baking
- **Procedure:** 1. Preheat oven to 180°C (350°F). 2. Mix flour, baking powder, ham, and cheese. 3. Whisk eggs, milk, and oil. 4. Combine wet and dry ingredients. 5. Divide into muffin tins. 6. Bake for 20 minutes. 7. Cool before serving.
- **Nutritional Values (per serving):** Calories: 220 kcal, Protein: 12g, Carbohydrates: 18g, Fat: 11g, Fiber: 2g, Sugars: 2g

Peanut Butter Oat Bars

- **Preparation Time:** 15 minutes (plus refrigeration)
- **Ingredients:** 1 cup rolled oats, 1/2 cup natural peanut butter, 1/4 cup maple syrup, 1/4 cup chopped nuts, 2 tablespoons chia seeds
- **Servings:** 6 bars
- **Cooking Method:** Refrigerating
- **Procedure:** 1. Mix all ingredients in a bowl. 2. Press mixture into a lined baking tray. 3. Refrigerate for 2 hours. 4. Cut into bars. 5. Store in an airtight container.
- **Nutritional Values (per serving):** Calories: 210 kcal, Protein: 6g, Carbohydrates: 22g, Fat: 11g, Fiber: 3g, Sugars: 10g

Savory Breakfast Rice Cakes

- **Preparation Time:** 10 minutes
- **Ingredients:** 2 rice cakes, 1 avocado (mashed), 1/4 cup canned tuna, 1 tablespoon lemon juice, salt and pepper to taste
- **Servings:** 2
- **Cooking Method:** Assembling
- **Procedure:** 1. Mix tuna, lemon juice, salt, and pepper. 2. Spread mashed avocado on rice cakes. 3. Top with tuna mixture. 4. Serve immediately.
- **Nutritional Values (per serving):** Calories: 240 kcal, Protein: 10g, Carbohydrates: 20g, Fat: 14g, Fiber: 6g, Sugars: 2g

Lactose-Free Cheese and Tomato Omelette Roll

- **Preparation Time:** 10 minutes
- **Ingredients:** 2 eggs, 1/4 cup grated lactose-free cheese, 1 small tomato (diced), 1 teaspoon olive oil, salt and pepper to taste
- **Servings:** 1
- **Cooking Method:** Frying
- **Procedure:** 1. Beat eggs with salt and pepper. 2. Heat oil in a skillet. 3. Pour in eggs, cook until set. 4. Sprinkle cheese and tomato. 5. Roll omelette. 6. Serve immediately.
- **Nutritional Values (per serving):** Calories: 220 kcal, Protein: 15g, Carbohydrates: 5g, Fat: 16g, Fiber: 1g, Sugars: 3g

Apple Cinnamon Overnight Oats

- **Preparation Time:** 8 hours (overnight soaking)
- **Ingredients:** 1/2 cup rolled oats, 1/2 cup almond milk, 1 small apple (grated), 1 teaspoon cinnamon, 1 tablespoon maple syrup
- **Servings:** 1
- **Cooking Method:** Soaking
- **Procedure:** 1. Combine oats, almond milk, cinnamon, and syrup in a jar. 2. Add grated apple. 3. Stir well and seal. 4. Refrigerate overnight. 5. Serve chilled.
- **Nutritional Values (per serving):** Calories: 270 kcal, Protein: 5g, Carbohydrates: 50g, Fat: 6g, Fiber: 6g, Sugars: 20g

Chapter 5: Satisfying Snacks and Appetizers

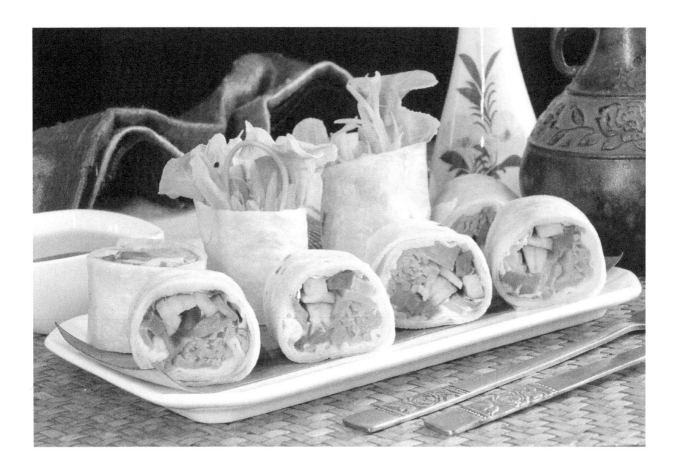

5.1. Light Bites for Busy Days

Almond Butter Rice Cake Toppers

- **Preparation Time:** 5 minutes
- **Ingredients:** 2 rice cakes, 2 tablespoons almond butter, 1/4 cup blueberries, 1 tablespoon sunflower seeds
- **Servings:** 2
- **Cooking Method:** Assembling
-

- **Procedure:** 1. Spread almond butter evenly on rice cakes. 2. Top with blueberries and sunflower seeds. 3. Serve immediately for a quick snack.
- **Nutritional Values (per serving):** Calories: 180 kcal, Protein: 4g, Carbohydrates: 20g, Fat: 10g, Fiber: 3g, Sugars: 5g

Carrot and Cucumber Hummus Rolls

- **Preparation Time:** 10 minutes
- **Ingredients:** 2 medium carrots (julienned), 1 cucumber (julienned), 1/4 cup hummus, 1 tablespoon lemon juice, pinch of salt
- **Servings:** 2
- **Cooking Method:** Rolling
- **Procedure:** 1. Mix hummus with lemon juice and salt. 2. Spread hummus on julienned carrots and cucumber strips. 3. Roll them up. 4. Serve chilled or immediately.
- **Nutritional Values (per serving):** Calories: 90 kcal, Protein: 3g, Carbohydrates: 14g, Fat: 3g, Fiber: 4g, Sugars: 6g

Spinach and Feta Cheese Stuffed Mushrooms

- **Preparation Time:** 20 minutes
- **Ingredients:** 6 button mushrooms (stems removed), 1/2 cup chopped spinach, 1/4 cup crumbled feta cheese, 1 teaspoon olive oil, salt and pepper to taste
- **Servings:** 2
- **Cooking Method:** Baking
- **Procedure:** 1. Preheat oven to 180°C (350°F). 2. Mix spinach, feta, salt, and pepper. 3. Stuff mixture into mushroom caps. 4. Drizzle with olive oil. 5. Bake for 15 minutes. 6. Serve warm.
- **Nutritional Values (per serving):** Calories: 120 kcal, Protein: 7g, Carbohydrates: 5g, Fat: 8g, Fiber: 1g, Sugars: 2g

Lactose-Free Greek Yogurt with Nuts and Honey

- **Preparation Time:** 5 minutes
- **Ingredients:** 1 cup lactose-free Greek yogurt, 2 tablespoons mixed nuts (chopped), 1 tablespoon honey
- **Servings:** 1
- **Cooking Method:** Mixing
- **Procedure:** 1. Place Greek yogurt in a bowl. 2. Top with chopped nuts. 3. Drizzle honey over the yogurt. 4. Serve immediately or chilled.
- **Nutritional Values (per serving):** Calories: 250 kcal, Protein: 15g, Carbohydrates: 20g, Fat: 12g, Fiber: 2g, Sugars: 18g

Gluten-Free Mini Veggie Quiches

- **Preparation Time:** 30 minutes
- **Ingredients:** 4 eggs, 1/2 cup chopped bell peppers, 1/2 cup chopped spinach, 1/4 cup grated cheddar cheese, 1/4 cup gluten-free flour, 1/4 cup lactose-free milk, salt and pepper to taste
- **Servings:** 4
- **Cooking Method:** Baking
- **Procedure:** 1. Preheat oven to 180°C (350°F). 2. Whisk eggs, milk, flour, salt, and pepper. 3. Stir in bell peppers, spinach, and cheese. 4. Pour into mini muffin tins. 5. Bake for 20 minutes. 6. Serve warm or cool.
- **Nutritional Values (per serving):** Calories: 150 kcal, Protein: 9g, Carbohydrates: 10g, Fat: 8g, Fiber: 1g, Sugars: 2g

Turkey and Avocado Roll-Ups

- **Preparation Time:** 10 minutes
- **Ingredients:** 4 slices turkey breast, 1 avocado (sliced), 1/4 cup arugula, 1 tablespoon Dijon mustard
- **Servings:** 2
- **Cooking Method:** Rolling
- **Procedure:** 1. Spread Dijon mustard over turkey slices. 2. Place avocado slices and arugula on turkey. 3. Roll up tightly. 4. Cut into bite-sized pieces. 5. Serve immediately.
- **Nutritional Values (per serving):** Calories: 200 kcal, Protein: 15g, Carbohydrates: 8g, Fat: 12g, Fiber: 4g, Sugars: 2g

5.2. Entertaining with Low-Fodmap Appetizers

Zesty Lemon-Garlic Shrimp Skewers

- **Preparation Time:** 20 minutes
- **Ingredients:** 200g shrimp (peeled), 1 tablespoon garlic-infused olive oil, 1 lemon (juice and zest), 1 teaspoon smoked paprika, fresh parsley for garnish
- **Servings:** 4
- **Cooking Method:** Grilling
- **Procedure:** 1. Marinate shrimp in lemon juice, zest, garlic-infused oil, and paprika for 10 minutes. 2. Thread shrimp onto skewers. 3. Grill for 3 minutes each side. 4. Garnish with parsley. 5. Serve hot.
- **Nutritional Values (per serving):** Calories: 120 kcal, Protein: 15g, Carbohydrates: 2g, Fat: 6g, Fiber: 0g, Sugars: 1g

Stuffed Cherry Tomatoes with Tuna Salad

- **Preparation Time:** 15 minutes
- **Ingredients:** 12 cherry tomatoes, 1 can tuna (drained), 2 tablespoons lactose-free mayonnaise, 1 teaspoon Dijon mustard, fresh dill for garnish
- **Servings:** 4
- **Cooking Method:** Assembling
- **Procedure:** 1. Cut tops off tomatoes and scoop out insides. 2. Mix tuna, mayonnaise, and mustard. 3. Stuff tomatoes with tuna mixture. 4. Garnish with dill. 5. Serve chilled.
- **Nutritional Values (per serving):** Calories: 80 kcal, Protein: 8g, Carbohydrates: 2g, Fat: 4g, Fiber: 1g, Sugars: 1g

Cucumber Rounds with Herbed Cream Cheese

- **Preparation Time:** 10 minutes
- **Ingredients:** 1 large cucumber, 1/2 cup lactose-free cream cheese, 1 tablespoon chopped chives, 1 tablespoon chopped dill, salt and pepper to taste
- **Servings:** 4
- **Cooking Method:** Assembling
- **Procedure:** 1. Slice cucumber into rounds. 2. Mix cream cheese with herbs, salt, and pepper. 3. Top cucumber rounds with herbed cream cheese. 4. Serve chilled.
- **Nutritional Values (per serving):** Calories: 70 kcal, Protein: 2g, Carbohydrates: 4g, Fat: 5g, Fiber: 1g, Sugars: 2g

Grilled Zucchini Roll-Ups

- **Preparation Time:** 20 minutes
- **Ingredients:** 2 zucchinis (sliced lengthwise), 1/4 cup roasted red peppers (sliced), 1/4 cup feta cheese (crumbled), 1 tablespoon olive oil, salt and pepper to taste
- **Servings:** 4
- **Cooking Method:** Grilling
- **Procedure:** 1. Brush zucchini slices with olive oil, season with salt and pepper. 2. Grill until tender. 3. Place red pepper and feta on zucchini slices. 4. Roll up and secure with toothpicks. 5. Serve warm or at room temperature.
- **Nutritional Values (per serving):** Calories: 90 kcal, Protein: 3g, Carbohydrates: 6g, Fat: 6g, Fiber: 1g, Sugars: 3g

Mini Bell Pepper Nachos

- **Preparation Time:** 20 minutes
- **Ingredients:** 6 mini bell peppers (halved and seeded), 1/2 cup cooked ground turkey, 1/4 cup lactose-free cheese (shredded), 1 tablespoon jalapeños (minced), salsa for serving
- **Servings:** 4
- **Cooking Method:** Baking

- **Procedure:** 1. Preheat oven to 200°C (400°F). 2. Fill pepper halves with ground turkey and jalapeños. 3. Top with cheese. 4. Bake for 10 minutes. 5. Serve with salsa.
- **Nutritional Values (per serving):** Calories: 120 kcal, Protein: 10g, Carbohydrates: 6g, Fat: 6g, Fiber: 1g, Sugars: 4g

Garlic-Infused Olive Tapenade on Gluten-Free Crackers

- **Preparation Time:** 15 minutes
- **Ingredients:** 1 cup black olives (pitted), 1 tablespoon garlic-infused olive oil, 1 teaspoon capers, 1 teaspoon lemon juice, gluten-free crackers for serving
- **Servings:** 4
- **Cooking Method:** Blending
- **Procedure:** 1. Blend olives, garlic-infused oil, capers, and lemon juice until smooth. 2. Spread tapenade on gluten-free crackers. 3. Serve immediately.
- **Nutritional Values (per serving):** Calories: 100 kcal, Protein: 1g, Carbohydrates: 10g, Fat: 6g, Fiber: 2g, Sugars: 0g

5.3. Nutritious Snacks for Energy Boost

Crunchy Peanut Butter Energy Balls

- **Preparation Time:** 15 minutes
- **Ingredients:** 1 cup rolled oats, 1/2 cup natural peanut butter, 1/4 cup honey, 2 tablespoons chia seeds, 1/4 cup dark chocolate chips (lactose-free)
- **Servings:** 10 balls

- **Cooking Method:** Mixing and Rolling
- **Procedure:** 1. Mix oats, peanut butter, honey, chia seeds, and chocolate chips. 2. Roll into small balls. 3. Chill in the refrigerator for 10 minutes. 4. Serve as an energy-boosting snack.
- **Nutritional Values (per serving):** Calories: 180 kcal, Protein: 5g, Carbohydrates: 20g, Fat: 10g, Fiber: 3g, Sugars: 10g

Fodmap-Friendly Trail Mix

- **Preparation Time:** 5 minutes
- **Ingredients:** 1/2 cup walnuts, 1/4 cup pumpkin seeds, 1/4 cup dried cranberries (low-Fodmap), 1/4 cup banana chips, pinch of sea salt
- **Servings:** 4
- **Cooking Method:** Mixing
- **Procedure:** 1. Combine walnuts, pumpkin seeds, cranberries, and banana chips in a bowl. 2. Sprinkle with sea salt. 3. Mix well and store in an airtight container. 4. Serve as a quick snack.
- **Nutritional Values (per serving):** Calories: 220 kcal, Protein: 5g, Carbohydrates: 15g, Fat: 16g, Fiber: 2g, Sugars: 8g

Avocado and Turkey Lettuce Wraps

- **Preparation Time:** 10 minutes
- **Ingredients:** 4 large lettuce leaves, 1 avocado (sliced), 100g turkey breast (sliced), 1 tablespoon lemon juice, salt and pepper to taste
- **Servings:** 2
- **Cooking Method:** Assembling
- **Procedure:** 1. Lay lettuce leaves flat. 2. Top with turkey and avocado slices. 3. Drizzle with lemon juice, season with salt and pepper. 4. Roll up and secure with toothpicks. 5. Serve fresh.
- **Nutritional Values (per serving):** Calories: 150 kcal, Protein: 15g, Carbohydrates: 8g, Fat: 8g, Fiber: 5g, Sugars: 1g

Greek Yogurt with Mixed Nuts and Honey

- **Preparation Time:** 5 minutes
- **Ingredients:** 1 cup lactose-free Greek yogurt, 1/4 cup mixed nuts (chopped), 2 tablespoons honey
- **Servings:** 1
- **Cooking Method:** Layering
- **Procedure:** 1. Spoon Greek yogurt into a bowl. 2. Top with chopped nuts. 3. Drizzle with honey. 4. Serve as a nourishing snack.
- **Nutritional Values (per serving):** Calories: 320 kcal, Protein: 18g, Carbohydrates: 30g, Fat: 16g, Fiber: 2g, Sugars: 25g

Roasted Chickpea Snack

- **Preparation Time:** 40 minutes
- **Ingredients:** 1 can chickpeas (drained and rinsed), 1 tablespoon olive oil, 1 teaspoon smoked paprika, salt to taste
- **Servings:** 4
- **Cooking Method:** Roasting
- **Procedure:** 1. Preheat oven to 200°C (400°F). 2. Toss chickpeas with olive oil, paprika, and salt. 3. Spread on baking sheet. 4. Roast for 30 minutes, stirring occasionally. 5. Cool before serving.
- **Nutritional Values (per serving):** Calories: 140 kcal, Protein: 6g, Carbohydrates: 15g, Fat: 6g, Fiber: 4g, Sugars: 2g

Lactose-Free Cheese and Grape Skewers

- **Preparation Time:** 10 minutes
- **Ingredients:** 12 grapes, 12 cubes lactose-free cheese, fresh basil leaves
- **Servings:** 4
- **Cooking Method:** Skewering
- **Procedure:** 1. Alternate grapes, cheese cubes, and basil leaves on skewers. 2. Chill in the refrigerator. 3. Serve as a refreshing and light snack.
- **Nutritional Values (per serving):** Calories: 100 kcal, Protein: 6g, Carbohydrates: 8g, Fat: 6g, Fiber: 1g, Sugars: 6g

Chapter 6: Wholesome Lunches

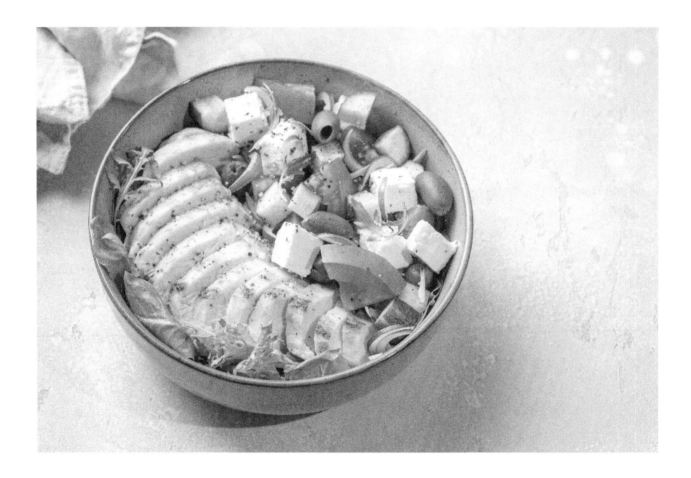

6.1. Quick Office-Friendly Lunches

Quinoa and Black Bean Salad

- **Preparation Time:** 20 minutes
- **Ingredients:** 1 cup cooked quinoa, 1/2 cup canned black beans (rinsed), 1/2 red bell pepper (diced), 2 tablespoons corn, 2 tablespoons cilantro (chopped), 1 tablespoon lime juice, 1 tablespoon olive oil, salt and pepper to taste
- **Servings:** 2
- **Cooking Method:** Mixing
- **Procedure:** 1. In a bowl, combine quinoa, black beans, bell pepper, and corn. 2. Add cilantro, lime juice, olive oil, salt, and pepper. 3. Toss to mix well. 4. Serve chilled or at room temperature.
- **Nutritional Values (per serving):** Calories: 250 kcal, Protein: 8g, Carbohydrates: 35g, Fat: 9g, Fiber: 7g, Sugars: 3g

Tuna and Avocado Wrap

- **Preparation Time:** 10 minutes
- **Ingredients:** 2 gluten-free tortillas, 1 can tuna (drained), 1 avocado (mashed), 1/4 cup mixed greens, 1 tablespoon mayonnaise (lactose-free), salt and pepper to taste
- **Servings:** 2
- **Cooking Method:** Assembling
- **Procedure:** 1. Spread mashed avocado on tortillas. 2. Mix tuna with mayonnaise, salt, and pepper. 3. Place tuna mixture and greens on tortillas. 4. Roll up and slice in half. 5. Serve immediately.
- **Nutritional Values (per serving):** Calories: 300 kcal, Protein: 20g, Carbohydrates: 25g, Fat: 15g, Fiber: 6g, Sugars: 2g

Zesty Chickpea and Cucumber Wrap

Preparation Time: 15 minutes
Ingredients: 1 cup canned chickpeas (rinsed and drained), 1 small cucumber (sliced), 2 whole wheat tortillas, 1 tablespoon Greek yogurt, 1 teaspoon lemon zest, salt, and ground cumin to taste
Servings: 2
Cooking Method: Assembling
Procedure: 1. Mash chickpeas in a bowl. 2. Mix in Greek yogurt, lemon zest, cumin, and salt. 3. Spread mixture onto tortillas. 4. Add cucumber slices and roll up the tortillas.
Nutritional Values (per serving): Calories: 280 kcal, Protein: 11g, Carbohydrates: 45g, Fat: 7g, Fiber: 8g, Sugars: 5g

Roasted Vegetable and Quinoa Bowl

- **Preparation Time:** 30 minutes
- **Ingredients:** 1 cup cooked quinoa, 1/2 cup roasted zucchini, 1/2 cup roasted bell peppers, 1/4 cup roasted cherry tomatoes, 1 tablespoon olive oil, 1 teaspoon balsamic vinegar, salt and pepper to taste
- **Servings:** 2
- **Cooking Method:** Roasting and Mixing
- **Procedure:** 1. Roast zucchini, bell peppers, and cherry tomatoes with olive oil, salt, and pepper. 2. Combine roasted vegetables with cooked quinoa. 3. Drizzle with balsamic vinegar. 4. Serve warm or at room temperature.
- **Nutritional Values (per serving):** Calories: 270 kcal, Protein: 8g, Carbohydrates: 35g, Fat: 12g, Fiber: 5g, Sugars: 4g

Spinach and Feta Stuffed Chicken Breast

- **Preparation Time:** 30 minutes
- **Ingredients:** 2 chicken breasts, 1/2 cup chopped spinach, 1/4 cup crumbled feta cheese (lactose-free), 1 tablespoon olive oil, salt and pepper to taste
- **Servings:** 2
- **Cooking Method:** Baking
- **Procedure:** 1. Preheat oven to 180°C (350°F). 2. Cut a pocket in each chicken breast. 3. Stuff with spinach and feta. 4. Season with salt and pepper. 5. Bake for 20 minutes. 6. Serve hot.
- **Nutritional Values (per serving):** Calories: 300 kcal, Protein: 30g, Carbohydrates: 2g, Fat: 18g, Fiber: 1g, Sugars: 1g

Rice Noodle Salad with Peanut Sauce

- **Preparation Time:** 20 minutes
- **Ingredients:** 1 cup cooked rice noodles, 1/2 cup shredded carrot, 1/2 cup shredded cabbage, 1/4 cup chopped cilantro, 2 tablespoons peanut butter, 1 tablespoon soy sauce (gluten-free), 1 teaspoon honey, 1 teaspoon lime juice
- **Servings:** 2
- **Cooking Method:** Mixing
- **Procedure:** 1. In a bowl, mix peanut butter, soy sauce, honey, and lime juice for the sauce. 2. Combine rice noodles, carrot, cabbage, and cilantro. 3. Toss with peanut sauce. 4. Serve chilled or at room temperature.
- **Nutritional Values (per serving):** Calories: 280 kcal, Protein: 6g, Carbohydrates: 40g, Fat: 10g, Fiber: 3g, Sugars: 5g

6.2. Hearty Home Lunches

Balsamic Glazed Chicken and Veggie Bowl

- **Preparation Time:** 25 minutes
- **Ingredients:** 2 chicken breasts, 1 cup broccoli florets, 1 red bell pepper (sliced), 2 tablespoons balsamic vinegar, 1 tablespoon olive oil, salt and pepper to taste
- **Servings:** 2
- **Cooking Method:** Baking and Sautéing
- **Procedure:** 1. Preheat oven to 200°C (400°F). 2. Season chicken with salt, pepper, and balsamic vinegar. 3. Bake chicken for 20 minutes. 4. Sauté broccoli and bell pepper in olive oil. 5. Slice chicken and serve with veggies.
- **Nutritional Values (per serving):** Calories: 300 kcal, Protein: 28g, Carbohydrates: 15g, Fat: 15g, Fiber: 3g, Sugars: 6g

Salmon and Avocado Salad

- **Preparation Time:** 15 minutes
- **Ingredients:** 1 cooked salmon fillet, 1 avocado (diced), 2 cups mixed greens, 1 tablespoon lemon juice, 1 tablespoon olive oil, salt and pepper to taste
- **Servings:** 2
- **Cooking Method:** Assembling
- **Procedure:** 1. Flake salmon fillet. 2. In a bowl, combine salmon, avocado, and mixed greens. 3. Dress with lemon juice, olive oil, salt, and pepper. 4. Toss and serve.
- **Nutritional Values (per serving):** Calories: 350 kcal, Protein: 24g, Carbohydrates: 12g, Fat: 25g, Fiber: 7g, Sugars: 2g

Turkey and Cheese Stuffed Bell Peppers

- **Preparation Time:** 30 minutes
- **Ingredients:** 2 bell peppers (halved and seeded), 200g ground turkey, 1/2 cup lactose-free cheese (shredded), 1 tablespoon tomato paste, salt and pepper to taste

- **Servings:** 2
- **Cooking Method:** Baking
- **Procedure:** 1. Preheat oven to 180°C (350°F). 2. Cook turkey with tomato paste, salt, and pepper. 3. Stuff bell peppers with turkey. 4. Top with cheese. 5. Bake for 15 minutes. 6. Serve hot.
- **Nutritional Values (per serving):** Calories: 280 kcal, Protein: 22g, Carbohydrates: 12g, Fat: 16g, Fiber: 3g, Sugars: 6g

Roasted Sweet Potato and Black Bean Bowls

Preparation Time: 35 minutes
Ingredients: 2 sweet potatoes (cubed), 1 cup black beans (cooked), 1 avocado (sliced), 1/4 cup red onion (diced), 1 teaspoon cumin, 2 tablespoons olive oil, salt, and chili powder
Servings: 2
Cooking Method: Roasting and Assembling
Procedure: 1. Preheat oven to 425°F (220°C). 2. Toss sweet potatoes with olive oil, cumin, chili powder, and salt. 3. Roast for 25 minutes. 4. Assemble bowls with sweet potatoes, black beans, avocado, and onion.
Nutritional Values (per serving):
Calories: 450 kcal, Protein: 10g, Carbohydrates: 55g, Fat: 22g, Fiber: 14g, Sugars: 9g

Gluten-Free Pasta Primavera

- **Preparation Time:** 20 minutes
- **Ingredients:** 2 cups gluten-free pasta, 1/2 cup zucchini (sliced), 1/2 cup cherry tomatoes (halved), 1/4 cup red onion (chopped), 2 tablespoons olive oil, 1 tablespoon garlic-infused oil, salt and pepper to taste
- **Servings:** 2
- **Cooking Method:** Boiling and Sautéing

- **Procedure:** 1. Cook pasta as per instructions. 2. Sauté vegetables in garlic-infused oil. 3. Mix cooked pasta with vegetables. 4. Drizzle with olive oil. 5. Season and serve.
- **Nutritional Values (per serving):** Calories: 320 kcal, Protein: 8g, Carbohydrates: 50g, Fat: 12g, Fiber: 3g, Sugars: 4g

Low-Fodmap Chicken Caesar Salad

- **Preparation Time:** 20 minutes
- **Ingredients:** 2 cups romaine lettuce (chopped), 1 grilled chicken breast (sliced), 1/4 cup grated parmesan cheese (lactose-free), 2 tablespoons Caesar dressing (low-Fodmap), croutons (gluten-free)
- **Servings:** 2
- **Cooking Method:** Assembling
- **Procedure:** 1. In a bowl, combine lettuce, chicken, and parmesan. 2. Add Caesar dressing and toss. 3. Top with gluten-free croutons. 4. Serve chilled.
- **Nutritional Values (per serving):** Calories: 250 kcal, Protein: 28g, Carbohydrates: 10g, Fat: 12g, Fiber: 2g, Sugars: 2g

Veggie and Quinoa Stuffed Acorn Squash

- **Preparation Time:** 45 minutes
- **Ingredients:** 2 acorn squashes (halved and seeded), 1 cup cooked quinoa, 1/2 cup diced carrots, 1/2 cup diced zucchini, 1/4 cup dried cranberries, 1 tablespoon olive oil, salt and pepper to taste
- **Servings:** 4
- **Cooking Method:** Baking and Stuffing

- **Procedure:** 1. Preheat oven to 180°C (350°F). 2. Brush squash with olive oil, season. 3. Bake squash for 25 minutes. 4. Mix quinoa, carrots, zucchini, and cranberries. 5. Stuff squash with quinoa mixture. 6. Bake for additional 15 minutes. 7. Serve warm.

- **Nutritional Values (per serving):** Calories: 240 kcal, Protein: 6g, Carbohydrates: 45g, Fat: 5g, Fiber: 6g, Sugars: 12g

6.3. Lunch Box Ideas for Everyone

Chicken and Veggie Pasta Salad

- **Preparation Time:** 20 minutes
- **Ingredients:** 2 cups cooked gluten-free pasta, 1 cup diced grilled chicken, 1/2 cup cherry tomatoes (halved), 1/2 cup cucumber (diced), 1/4 cup Italian dressing (low-Fodmap), salt and pepper to taste
- **Servings:** 2
- **Cooking Method:** Mixing

- **Procedure:** 1. In a large bowl, mix pasta, chicken, tomatoes, and cucumber. 2. Toss with Italian dressing. 3. Season with salt and pepper. 4. Refrigerate until serving.
- **Nutritional Values (per serving):** Calories: 350 kcal, Protein: 20g, Carbohydrates: 40g, Fat: 12g, Fiber: 2g, Sugars: 4g

Tofu and Veggie Stir-Fry

- **Preparation Time:** 15 minutes
- **Ingredients:** 200g firm tofu (cubed), 1 cup mixed bell peppers (sliced), 1/2 cup snow peas, 2 tablespoons soy sauce (gluten-free), 1 tablespoon sesame oil, 1 teaspoon ginger (minced)
- **Servings:** 2
- **Cooking Method:** Stir-frying
- **Procedure:** 1. Heat sesame oil in a pan. 2. Add tofu and cook until golden. 3. Add vegetables, ginger, and soy sauce. 4. Stir-fry for 5 minutes. 5. Serve hot or cold.
- **Nutritional Values (per serving):** Calories: 220 kcal, Protein: 12g, Carbohydrates: 10g, Fat: 15g, Fiber: 3g, Sugars: 4g

Quinoa Veggie Mason Jar Salad

- **Preparation Time:** 15 minutes
- **Ingredients:** 1 cup cooked quinoa, 1/2 cup cherry tomatoes (halved), 1/2 cup cucumber (diced), 1/4 cup red onion (chopped), 1/4 cup feta cheese (lactose-free), 2 tablespoons balsamic vinaigrette
- **Servings:** 2

- **Cooking Method:** Layering
- **Procedure:** 1. In a mason jar, layer quinoa, tomatoes, cucumber, onion, and feta. 2. Top with balsamic vinaigrette. 3. Seal and refrigerate. 4. Shake before serving.
- **Nutritional Values (per serving):** Calories: 320 kcal, Protein: 10g, Carbohydrates: 45g, Fat: 12g, Fiber: 5g, Sugars: 6g

Teriyaki Tofu and Broccoli Rice Bowl

Preparation Time: 30 minutes
Ingredients: 1 cup tofu (cubed), 1 cup broccoli florets, 1 cup cooked brown rice, 2 tablespoons teriyaki sauce, 1 tablespoon sesame oil, sesame seeds, and green onions for garnish
Servings: 2
Cooking Method: Stir-frying
Procedure: 1. Stir-fry tofu in sesame oil until golden. 2. Add broccoli and teriyaki sauce, cook until tender. 3. Serve over brown rice, garnish with sesame seeds and green onions.
Nutritional Values (per serving): Calories: 350 kcal, Protein: 15g, Carbohydrates: 45g, Fat: 15g, Fiber: 5g, Sugars: 8g

Turkey Lettuce Wraps

- **Preparation Time:** 15 minutes
- **Ingredients:** 200g ground turkey, 1 tablespoon garlic-infused oil, 4 lettuce leaves, 1/4 cup shredded carrots, 1 tablespoon hoisin sauce (gluten-free), fresh cilantro for garnish
- **Servings:** 2
- **Cooking Method:** Sautéing

- **Procedure:** 1. Cook turkey in garlic-infused oil. 2. Stir in hoisin sauce. 3. Place turkey mixture on lettuce leaves. 4. Top with carrots and cilantro. 5. Roll and serve.
- **Nutritional Values (per serving):** Calories: 250 kcal, Protein: 25g, Carbohydrates: 10g, Fat: 12g, Fiber: 2g, Sugars: 5g

Roasted Sweet Potato and Chickpea Bowl

- **Preparation Time:** 30 minutes
- **Ingredients:** 1 sweet potato (cubed), 1/2 cup canned chickpeas (rinsed), 1 tablespoon olive oil, 1/2 teaspoon smoked paprika, 1 cup spinach, 2 tablespoons tahini sauce
- **Servings:** 2
- **Cooking Method:** Roasting
- **Procedure:** 1. Preheat oven to 200°C (400°F). 2. Toss sweet potato and chickpeas with olive oil and paprika. 3. Roast for 25 minutes. 4. Serve over spinach, drizzle with tahini.
- **Nutritional Values (per serving):** Calories: 330 kcal, Protein: 8g, Carbohydrates: 45g, Fat: 15g, Fiber: 9g, Sugars: 10g

Mediterranean Tuna Salad Pita

- **Preparation Time:** 10 minutes
- **Ingredients:** 1 can tuna (drained), 1/4 cup diced cucumber, 1/4 cup diced tomato, 1/4 cup chopped olives, 2 tablespoons Greek yogurt (lactose-free), 2 pita breads (gluten-free), fresh parsley for garnish
- **Servings:** 2

- **Cooking Method:** Mixing and Assembling
- **Procedure:** 1. Mix tuna, cucumber, tomato, olives, and Greek yogurt. 2. Fill pita breads with tuna salad. 3. Garnish with parsley. 4. Serve chilled or at room temperature.
- **Nutritional Values (per serving):** Calories: 320 kcal, Protein: 20g, Carbohydrates: 40g, Fat: 9g, Fiber: 5g, Sugars: 4g

Chapter 7: Nourishing Dinners

7.1. Family-Friendly Meals

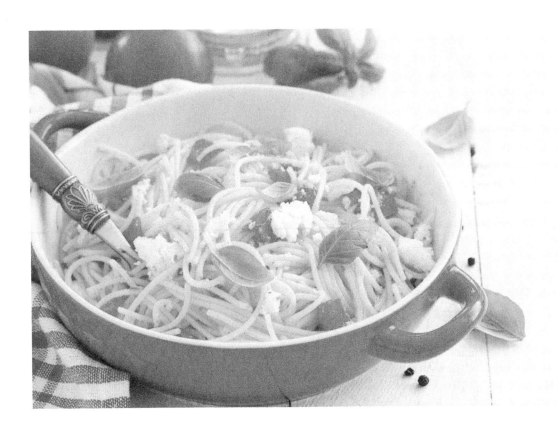

Baked Lemon-Garlic Chicken with Veggies

- **Preparation Time:** 35 minutes
- **Ingredients:** 4 chicken thighs, 1 lemon (juiced), 2 tablespoons garlic-infused olive oil, 1 cup green beans, 1 cup cherry tomatoes, salt and pepper to taste
- **Servings:** 4
- **Cooking Method:** Baking
- **Procedure:** 1. Marinate chicken in lemon juice, garlic-infused oil, salt, and pepper. 2. Arrange chicken, green beans, and tomatoes on a baking tray. 3. Bake at 200°C (400°F) for 30 minutes. 4. Serve hot.
- **Nutritional Values (per serving):** Calories: 280 kcal, Protein: 22g, Carbohydrates: 6g, Fat: 18g, Fiber: 2g, Sugars: 3g

Fodmap-Friendly Beef Stir-Fry

- **Preparation Time:** 20 minutes
- **Ingredients:** 400g sliced beef, 1 cup bell peppers (sliced), 1/2 cup carrot (julienne), 2 tablespoons tamari sauce, 1 tablespoon sesame oil, 1 teaspoon ginger (minced)
- **Servings:** 4
- **Cooking Method:** Stir-frying
- **Procedure:** 1. Heat sesame oil in a pan. 2. Cook beef until browned. 3. Add vegetables, ginger, and tamari sauce. 4. Stir-fry for 5 minutes. 5. Serve with rice if desired.
- **Nutritional Values (per serving):** Calories: 250 kcal, Protein: 25g, Carbohydrates: 8g, Fat: 12g, Fiber: 1g, Sugars: 3g

Vegetable Stir-Fry with Brown Rice

Preparation Time: 25 minutes
Ingredients: 2 cups mixed vegetables (broccoli, bell pepper, carrot, snap peas), 1 cup brown rice (cooked), 2 tablespoons soy sauce, 1 tablespoon sesame oil, 1 garlic clove (minced), 1 teaspoon ginger (grated)
Servings: 2
Cooking Method: Stir-frying
Procedure: 1. Heat sesame oil in a pan, add garlic and ginger, sauté for 1 minute. 2. Add vegetables, stir-fry until tender. 3. Add cooked rice and soy sauce, mix well.
Nutritional Values (per serving): Calories: 300 kcal, Protein: 6g, Carbohydrates: 45g, Fat: 10g, Fiber: 4g, Sugars: 5g

Gluten-Free Spaghetti with Tomato Basil Sauce

- **Preparation Time:** 30 minutes
- **Ingredients:** 2 cups gluten-free spaghetti, 1 cup tomato sauce (low-Fodmap), 1/4 cup fresh basil (chopped), 1 tablespoon olive oil, grated Parmesan cheese (lactose-free), salt and pepper to taste
- **Servings:** 4
- **Cooking Method:** Boiling and Simmering
- **Procedure:** 1. Cook spaghetti as per package instructions. 2. Heat tomato sauce with olive oil, basil, salt, and pepper. 3. Toss cooked spaghetti with sauce. 4. Top with Parmesan cheese. 5. Serve warm.
- **Nutritional Values (per serving):** Calories: 320 kcal, Protein: 8g, Carbohydrates: 50g, Fat: 10g, Fiber: 2g, Sugars: 3g

Maple-Glazed Salmon with Steamed Vegetables

- **Preparation Time:** 20 minutes
- **Ingredients:** 4 salmon fillets, 2 tablespoons maple syrup, 1 tablespoon soy sauce (gluten-free), 2 cups mixed vegetables (carrots, broccoli, zucchini), salt and pepper to taste
- **Servings:** 4
- **Cooking Method:** Baking and Steaming
- **Procedure:** 1. Mix maple syrup and soy sauce. 2. Glaze salmon with mixture. 3. Bake at 200°C (400°F) for 15 minutes. 4. Steam vegetables. 5. Serve salmon with steamed veggies.
- **Nutritional Values (per serving):** Calories: 300 kcal, Protein: 23g, Carbohydrates: 12g, Fat: 18g, Fiber: 3g, Sugars: 7g

Turkey Meatball and Veggie Pasta Bake

- **Preparation Time:** 45 minutes
- **Ingredients:** 500g ground turkey, 2 cups gluten-free pasta, 1 cup tomato sauce (low-Fodmap), 1/2 cup zucchini (diced), 1/2 cup bell peppers (diced), 1/4 cup grated cheese (lactose-free), 1 egg, herbs to taste
- **Servings:** 4
- **Cooking Method:** Baking
- **Procedure:** 1. Mix turkey, egg, and herbs. 2. Form into meatballs. 3. Cook pasta; mix with sauce, zucchini, and bell peppers. 4. Add meatballs to pasta mixture. 5. Top with cheese. 6. Bake at 180°C (350°F) for 30 minutes. 7. Serve hot.
- **Nutritional Values (per serving):** Calories: 400 kcal, Protein: 28g, Carbohydrates: 40g, Fat: 16g, Fiber: 4g, Sugars: 6g

7.2. Romantic Dinner Recipes

Seared Scallops with Lemon-Herb Butter

- **Preparation Time:** 20 minutes
- **Ingredients:** 8 large sea scallops, 2 tablespoons unsalted butter, 1 tablespoon fresh lemon juice, 1 teaspoon chopped parsley, 1 teaspoon chopped basil, salt and pepper to taste
- **Servings:** 2
- **Cooking Method:** Searing
- **Procedure:** 1. Season scallops with salt and pepper. 2. Sear scallops in a pan for 2 minutes each side. 3. Melt butter in the pan, add lemon juice, parsley, and basil. 4. Spoon butter over scallops. 5. Serve immediately.
- **Nutritional Values (per serving):** Calories: 200 kcal, Protein: 14g, Carbohydrates: 3g, Fat: 15g, Fiber: 0g, Sugars: 0g

Grilled Salmon with Asparagus and Dill Sauce

- **Preparation Time:** 30 minutes
- **Ingredients:** 2 salmon fillets, 1 bunch asparagus, 2 tablespoons olive oil, 1/4 cup dill sauce (low-Fodmap), salt and pepper to taste
- **Servings:** 2
- **Cooking Method:** Grilling
- **Procedure:** 1. Brush salmon and asparagus with olive oil, season. 2. Grill for 5-7 minutes per side. 3. Serve with dill sauce.
- **Nutritional Values (per serving):** Calories: 310 kcal, Protein: 23g, Carbohydrates: 4g, Fat: 23g, Fiber: 2g, Sugars: 2g

Caprese Stuffed Chicken Breast

- **Preparation Time:** 40 minutes
- **Ingredients:** 2 chicken breasts, 1/4 cup sliced mozzarella (lactose-free), 1 tomato (sliced), fresh basil leaves, 1 tablespoon olive oil, balsamic glaze (low-Fodmap), salt and pepper to taste

- **Servings:** 2
- **Cooking Method:** Baking
- **Procedure:** 1. Preheat oven to 180°C (350°F). 2. Cut a pocket in each chicken breast. 3. Stuff with mozzarella, tomato, basil. 4. Season, drizzle with oil. 5. Bake for 25 minutes. 6. Drizzle with balsamic glaze.
- **Nutritional Values (per serving):** Calories: 280 kcal, Protein: 30g, Carbohydrates: 4g, Fat: 15g, Fiber: 1g, Sugars: 2g

Roasted Vegetable and Quinoa Medley

- **Preparation Time:** 35 minutes
- **Ingredients:** 1 cup quinoa, 1/2 cup chopped bell peppers, 1/2 cup cherry tomatoes, 1/2 cup zucchini (cubed), 2 tablespoons olive oil, 1 teaspoon dried thyme, salt and pepper to taste
- **Servings:** 2
- **Cooking Method:** Roasting and Boiling

- **Procedure:** 1. Cook quinoa as per instructions. 2. Toss vegetables with oil, thyme, salt, pepper. 3. Roast at 200°C (400°F) for 20 minutes. 4. Mix with quinoa. 5. Serve warm.
- **Nutritional Values (per serving):** Calories: 320 kcal, Protein: 10g, Carbohydrates: 45g, Fat: 12g, Fiber: 5g, Sugars: 4g

Herb-Crusted Rack of Lamb

- **Preparation Time:** 45 minutes
- **Ingredients:** 1 rack of lamb (8 ribs), 2 tablespoons Dijon mustard, 1/4 cup breadcrumbs (gluten-free), 1 tablespoon chopped rosemary, 1 tablespoon chopped thyme, olive oil, salt and pepper to taste
- **Servings:** 2
- **Cooking Method:** Roasting
- **Procedure:** 1. Preheat oven to 200°C (400°F). 2. Rub lamb with mustard. 3. Mix breadcrumbs, herbs, oil, salt, pepper. 4. Coat lamb with breadcrumb mixture. 5. Roast for 20-25 minutes. 6. Let rest, then slice.
- **Nutritional Values (per serving):** Calories: 420 kcal, Protein: 35g, Carbohydrates: 12g, Fat: 26g, Fiber: 1g, Sugars: 1g

7.3. Dinner Parties on a Low-Fodmap Diet

Citrus-Infused Baked Cod with Herb Salad

- **Preparation Time:** 30 minutes
- **Ingredients:** 4 cod fillets, 1 lemon (sliced), 1 orange (sliced), mixed fresh herbs (parsley, dill, chives), 2 tablespoons olive oil, salt and pepper to taste
- **Servings:** 4
- **Cooking Method:** Baking

- **Procedure:** 1. Preheat oven to 180°C (350°F). 2. Place cod on baking sheet, top with citrus slices, drizzle with oil, season. 3. Bake for 20 minutes. 4. Serve with a fresh herb salad.
- **Nutritional Values (per serving):** Calories: 200 kcal, Protein: 22g, Carbohydrates: 5g, Fat: 10g, Fiber: 1g, Sugars: 2g

Roasted Vegetable and Quinoa Risotto

- **Preparation Time:** 40 minutes
- **Ingredients:** 1 cup quinoa, 2 cups vegetable broth (low-Fodmap), 1 cup roasted vegetables (zucchini, bell pepper), 1/4 cup Parmesan cheese (lactose-free), 1 tablespoon olive oil, salt and pepper to taste
- **Servings:** 4
- **Cooking Method:** Roasting and Simmering
- **Procedure:** 1. Cook quinoa in broth until tender. 2. Stir in roasted vegetables, cheese, oil. 3. Season with salt and pepper. 4. Serve warm.
- **Nutritional Values (per serving):** Calories: 310 kcal, Protein: 12g, Carbohydrates: 45g, Fat: 10g, Fiber: 4g, Sugars: 3g

Grilled Steak with Chimichurri Sauce

- **Preparation Time:** 25 minutes
- **Ingredients:** 4 steak cuts (sirloin or ribeye), 1/2 cup chimichurri sauce (low-Fodmap), 2 tablespoons olive oil, salt and pepper to taste
- **Servings:** 4
- **Cooking Method:** Grilling
- **Procedure:** 1. Season steaks with salt, pepper, oil. 2. Grill to desired doneness. 3. Serve with chimichurri sauce.
- **Nutritional Values (per serving):** Calories: 350 kcal, Protein: 30g, Carbohydrates: 2g, Fat: 25g, Fiber: 0g, Sugars: 0g

Lemon-Thyme Roasted Chicken with Potatoes

- **Preparation Time:** 60 minutes
- **Ingredients:** 1 whole chicken, 4 potatoes (cubed), 2 tablespoons thyme leaves, 1 lemon (sliced), 3 tablespoons olive oil, salt and pepper to taste
- **Servings:** 4-6
- **Cooking Method:** Roasting
- **Procedure:** 1. Preheat oven to 200°C (390°F). 2. Season chicken, stuff with lemon slices, coat with oil, thyme. 3. Surround with potatoes. 4. Roast for 50 minutes. 5. Serve hot.
- **Nutritional Values (per serving):** Calories: 420 kcal, Protein: 35g, Carbohydrates: 20g, Fat: 22g, Fiber: 3g, Sugars: 1g

Herb-Crusted Rack of Lamb with Mint Pesto

- **Preparation Time:** 45 minutes
- **Ingredients:** 1 rack of lamb (8 ribs), 1/4 cup breadcrumbs (gluten-free), 2 tablespoons mixed herbs (rosemary, thyme), 1/4 cup mint pesto (low-Fodmap), 2 tablespoons olive oil, salt and pepper to taste
- **Servings:** 2-3
- **Cooking Method:** Roasting
- **Procedure:** 1. Preheat oven to 220°C (430°F). 2. Mix breadcrumbs, herbs, oil, season lamb. 3. Coat lamb with breadcrumb mixture. 4. Roast for 20 minutes. 5. Serve with mint pesto.
- **Nutritional Values (per serving):** Calories: 500 kcal, Protein: 40g, Carbohydrates: 15g, Fat: 32g, Fiber: 2g, Sugars: 2g

Chapter 8: Comforting Soups and Salads

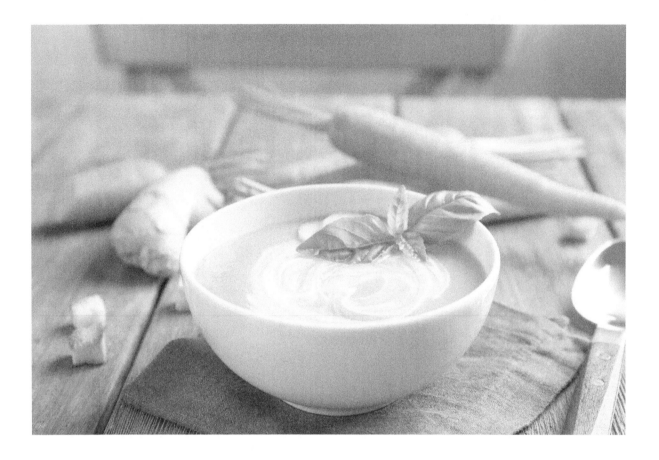

8.1. Warm and Cozy Soups

- **Preparation Time:** 30 minutes
- **Ingredients:** 4 large carrots (chopped), 1 tablespoon grated ginger, 2 cups low-Fodmap vegetable broth, 1 cup lactose-free cream, 1 teaspoon olive oil, salt and pepper to taste
- **Servings:** 4
- **Cooking Method:** Simmering
- **Procedure:** 1. Sauté carrots and ginger in oil for 5 minutes. 2. Add broth, simmer until carrots are tender. 3. Blend until smooth. 4. Stir in cream, season. 5. Serve warm.
- **Nutritional Values (per serving):** Calories: 150 kcal, Protein: 2g, Carbohydrates: 18g, Fat: 8g, Fiber: 4g, Sugars: 6g

Rustic Pumpkin and Thyme Soup

- **Preparation Time:** 45 minutes
- **Ingredients:** 2 cups pumpkin puree, 3 cups low-Fodmap chicken broth, 1 teaspoon dried thyme, 2 tablespoons olive oil, salt and pepper to taste
- **Servings:** 4
- **Cooking Method:** Blending and Simmering
- **Procedure:** 1. Heat oil, add thyme, cook for 1 minute. 2. Add pumpkin, broth, simmer 30 minutes. 3. Blend until smooth. 4. Season with salt, pepper. 5. Serve hot.
- **Nutritional Values (per serving):** Calories: 120 kcal, Protein: 2g, Carbohydrates: 15g, Fat: 6g, Fiber: 4g, Sugars: 5g

Hearty Beef and Potato Stew

- **Preparation Time:** 60 minutes
- **Ingredients:** 1 lb beef stew meat, 3 large potatoes (cubed), 4 cups low-Fodmap beef broth, 1 teaspoon rosemary, 2 tablespoons olive oil, salt and pepper to taste
- **Servings:** 4
- **Cooking Method:** Slow Cooking
- **Procedure:** 1. Brown beef in oil. 2. Add potatoes, broth, rosemary. 3. Simmer for 45 minutes. 4. Season and serve.
- **Nutritional Values (per serving):** Calories: 350 kcal, Protein: 28g, Carbohydrates: 30g, Fat: 15g, Fiber: 4g, Sugars: 2g

Tomato Basil Bisque

- **Preparation Time:** 30 minutes
- **Ingredients:** 2 cans diced tomatoes (low-Fodmap), 1 cup lactose-free milk, 1/4 cup chopped fresh basil, 1 tablespoon olive oil, salt and pepper to taste
- **Servings:** 4
- **Cooking Method:** Blending and Simmering
- **Procedure:** 1. Sauté tomatoes in oil for 5 minutes. 2. Add basil, simmer for 15 minutes. 3. Blend with milk until smooth. 4. Season and serve.
- **Nutritional Values (per serving):** Calories: 110 kcal, Protein: 3g, Carbohydrates: 12g, Fat: 6g, Fiber: 2g, Sugars: 6g

Lentil and Spinach Soup

- **Preparation Time:** 45 minutes
- **Ingredients:** 1 cup dried lentils, 3 cups low-Fodmap vegetable broth, 2 cups fresh spinach, 1 teaspoon cumin, 2 tablespoons olive oil, salt and pepper to taste
- **Servings:** 4
- **Cooking Method:** Simmering
- **Procedure:** 1. Cook lentils in broth until tender. 2. Add spinach, cumin, simmer 10 minutes. 3. Drizzle with olive oil, season. 4. Serve hot.
- **Nutritional Values (per serving):** Calories: 220 kcal, Protein: 15g, Carbohydrates: 30g, Fat: 6g, Fiber: 15g, Sugars: 3g

8.2. Fresh and Flavorful Salads

Citrus Quinoa and Mixed Greens Salad

- **Preparation Time:** 20 minutes
- **Ingredients:** 1 cup cooked quinoa, 1/2 cup sliced oranges, 2 cups mixed greens, 1/4 cup chopped walnuts, 1/4 cup diced cucumber, dressing of olive oil and lemon juice, salt and pepper to taste
- **Servings:** 2
- **Cooking Method:** Tossing
- **Procedure:** 1. Combine quinoa, oranges, greens, cucumber, and walnuts. 2. Whisk together olive oil, lemon juice, salt, and pepper. 3. Toss the salad with the dressing. 4. Serve chilled.
- **Nutritional Values (per serving):** Calories: 280 kcal, Protein: 8g, Carbohydrates: 30g, Fat: 15g, Fiber: 5g, Sugars: 6g

Beetroot and Feta Cheese Salad

- **Preparation Time:** 15 minutes
- **Ingredients:** 2 cups diced cooked beetroot, 1/2 cup crumbled feta cheese, 2 tablespoons pine nuts, 2 cups arugula, dressing of balsamic vinegar and olive oil, salt and pepper to taste
- **Servings:** 2
- **Cooking Method:** Mixing
- **Procedure:** 1. Combine beetroot, feta, arugula, and pine nuts in a bowl. 2. Drizzle with balsamic vinegar and olive oil. 3. Season with salt and pepper. 4. Toss gently and serve.

- **Nutritional Values (per serving):** Calories: 250 kcal, Protein: 7g, Carbohydrates: 18g, Fat: 18g, Fiber: 4g, Sugars: 12g

Avocado and Spinach Salad with Lemon Dressing

- **Preparation Time:** 10 minutes
- **Ingredients:** 1 ripe avocado (sliced), 2 cups baby spinach, 1/4 cup slivered almonds, dressing of lemon juice and olive oil, salt and pepper to taste
- **Servings:** 2
- **Cooking Method:** Tossing
- **Procedure:** 1. Place spinach and avocado slices in a bowl. 2. Top with almonds. 3. Combine lemon juice and olive oil for dressing. 4. Drizzle over salad, season, and serve.
- **Nutritional Values (per serving):** Calories: 300 kcal, Protein: 5g, Carbohydrates: 15g, Fat: 27g, Fiber: 7g, Sugars: 2g

Grilled Chicken and Romaine Salad

- **Preparation Time:** 30 minutes
- **Ingredients:** 1 grilled chicken breast (sliced), 3 cups romaine lettuce, 1/4 cup cherry tomatoes, 2 tablespoons grated Parmesan, dressing of lemon juice and olive oil, salt and pepper to taste
- **Servings:** 2
- **Cooking Method:** Grilling and Tossing

- **Procedure:** 1. Grill chicken, slice. 2. Toss lettuce, tomatoes, and chicken. 3. Sprinkle with Parmesan. 4. Combine lemon juice and olive oil, drizzle over salad. 5. Season and serve.
- **Nutritional Values (per serving):** Calories: 250 kcal, Protein: 28g, Carbohydrates: 6g, Fat: 12g, Fiber: 3g, Sugars: 3g

Walnut, Pear, and Gorgonzola Salad

- **Preparation Time:** 15 minutes
- **Ingredients:** 2 cups mixed salad greens, 1 ripe pear (sliced), 1/4 cup crumbled Gorgonzola cheese, 1/4 cup chopped walnuts, dressing of apple cider vinegar and olive oil, salt and pepper to taste
- **Servings:** 2
- **Cooking Method:** Mixing
- **Procedure:** 1. Combine greens, pear slices, Gorgonzola, and walnuts. 2. Whisk together apple cider vinegar and olive oil. 3. Toss salad with dressing. 4. Season with salt and pepper, serve immediately.
- **Nutritional Values (per serving):** Calories: 280 kcal, Protein: 7g, Carbohydrates: 15g, Fat: 22g, Fiber: 4g, Sugars: 9g

8.3. Dressings and Toppings

Creamy Avocado Dressing

- **Preparation Time:** 10 minutes
- **Ingredients:** 1 ripe avocado, 1/4 cup Greek yogurt, 2 tablespoons olive oil, 1 tablespoon lime juice, 1 garlic clove, salt, and pepper to taste
- **Servings:** 4
- **Cooking Method:** Blending
- **Procedure:** 1. Blend avocado, yogurt, olive oil, lime juice, and garlic until smooth. 2. Season with salt and pepper. 3. Refrigerate until serving.
- **Nutritional Values (per serving):** Calories: 120 kcal, Protein: 2g, Carbohydrates: 6g, Fat: 10g, Fiber: 3g, Sugars: 1g

Honey Mustard Vinaigrette

- **Preparation Time:** 5 minutes
- **Ingredients:** 3 tablespoons olive oil, 1 tablespoon apple cider vinegar, 2 teaspoons honey, 1 teaspoon Dijon mustard, salt, and pepper to taste
- **Servings:** 4
- **Cooking Method:** Whisking
- **Procedure:** 1. Whisk together olive oil, vinegar, honey, and mustard. 2. Season with salt and pepper. 3. Store in the refrigerator.
- **Nutritional Values (per serving):** Calories: 90 kcal, Protein: 0g, Carbohydrates: 4g, Fat: 8g, Fiber: 0g, Sugars: 4g

Basil Pesto Topping

- **Preparation Time:** 15 minutes
- **Ingredients:** 2 cups fresh basil leaves, 1/4 cup pine nuts, 1/2 cup grated Parmesan cheese, 2 garlic cloves, 1/2 cup olive oil, salt, and pepper to taste
- **Servings:** 4
- **Cooking Method:** Blending
- **Procedure:** 1. Blend basil, pine nuts, Parmesan, and garlic. 2. Gradually add olive oil while blending. 3. Season with salt and pepper. 4. Refrigerate until use.
- **Nutritional Values (per serving):** Calories: 250 kcal, Protein: 6g, Carbohydrates: 2g, Fat: 25g, Fiber: 1g, Sugars: 0g

Tangy Lemon Tahini Dressing

- **Preparation Time:** 10 minutes
- **Ingredients:** 1/4 cup tahini, 1/4 cup water, 2 tablespoons lemon juice, 1 garlic clove, salt, and pepper to taste
- **Servings:** 4
- **Cooking Method:** Whisking
- **Procedure:** 1. Whisk together tahini, water, and lemon juice. 2. Add minced garlic. 3. Season with salt and pepper. 4. Store chilled.
- **Nutritional Values (per serving):** Calories: 100 kcal, Protein: 3g, Carbohydrates: 3g, Fat: 9g, Fiber: 1g, Sugars: 0g

Balsamic Reduction

- **Preparation Time:** 20 minutes
- **Ingredients:** 1 cup balsamic vinegar, 2 tablespoons honey
- **Servings:** 4
- **Cooking Method:** Simmering
- **Procedure:** 1. Combine vinegar and honey in a saucepan. 2. Simmer until reduced by half. 3. Cool and refrigerate.
- **Nutritional Values (per serving):** Calories: 80 kcal, Protein: 0g, Carbohydrates: 17g, Fat: 0g, Fiber: 0g, Sugars: 15g

Chapter 9: Tasty Side Dishes

9.1. Vegetable-Based Sides

Roasted Garlic Green Beans

- **Preparation Time:** 20 minutes
- **Ingredients:** 2 cups green beans, 1 tablespoon olive oil, 3 garlic cloves, minced, salt, and pepper to taste
- **Servings:** 4
- **Cooking Method:** Roasting
- **Procedure:** 1. Toss green beans with olive oil and garlic. 2. Spread on a baking sheet. 3. Roast at 400°F for 15 minutes. 4. Season with salt and pepper. 5. Serve warm.
- **Nutritional Values (per serving):** Calories: 50 kcal, Protein: 2g, Carbohydrates: 6g, Fat: 2.5g, Fiber: 2g, Sugars: 1g

Honey-Glazed Carrot Coins

- **Preparation Time:** 25 minutes
- **Ingredients:** 3 large carrots, sliced, 2 tablespoons honey, 1 tablespoon butter, salt, and pepper to taste
- **Servings:** 4
- **Cooking Method:** Sautéing
- **Procedure:** 1. Sauté carrots in butter until tender. 2. Add honey, cook for 5 minutes. 3. Season with salt and pepper. 4. Serve hot.
- **Nutritional Values (per serving):** Calories: 90 kcal, Protein: 1g, Carbohydrates: 15g, Fat: 3g, Fiber: 2g, Sugars: 11g

Balsamic Brussel Sprouts

- **Preparation Time:** 30 minutes
- **Ingredients:** 2 cups Brussels sprouts, halved, 2 tablespoons balsamic vinegar, 1 tablespoon olive oil, salt and pepper to taste
- **Servings:** 4
- **Cooking Method:** Roasting
- **Procedure:** 1. Toss Brussels sprouts with olive oil and vinegar. 2. Roast at 375°F for 25 minutes. 3. Season with salt and pepper. 4. Serve warm.
- **Nutritional Values (per serving):** Calories: 80 kcal, Protein: 3g, Carbohydrates: 10g, Fat: 4g, Fiber: 3g, Sugars: 3g

Spicy Cauliflower Steaks

- **Preparation Time:** 35 minutes
- **Ingredients:** 1 large cauliflower, sliced into steaks, 2 tablespoons olive oil, 1 teaspoon paprika, 1/2 teaspoon chili powder, salt, and pepper to taste
- **Servings:** 4
- **Cooking Method:** Baking
- **Procedure:** 1. Brush cauliflower steaks with olive oil. 2. Sprinkle with spices. 3. Bake at 400°F for 30 minutes. 4. Season with salt and pepper. 5. Serve hot.
- **Nutritional Values (per serving):** Calories: 120 kcal, Protein: 4g, Carbohydrates: 11g, Fat: 7g, Fiber: 3g, Sugars: 4g

Lemon Herb Zucchini Ribbons

- **Preparation Time:** 15 minutes
- **Ingredients:** 3 zucchinis, sliced into ribbons, 2 tablespoons lemon juice, 1 tablespoon olive oil, 1 teaspoon mixed herbs, salt, and pepper to taste
- **Servings:** 4
- **Cooking Method:** Sautéing
- **Procedure:** 1. Sauté zucchini ribbons in olive oil. 2. Add lemon juice and herbs. 3. Cook for 5 minutes. 4. Season with salt and pepper. 5. Serve warm.
- **Nutritional Values (per serving):** Calories: 50 kcal, Protein: 2g, Carbohydrates: 4g, Fat: 3g, Fiber: 1g, Sugars: 2g

9.2. Creative Carb Alternatives

Cauliflower Rice Pilaf

- **Preparation Time:** 20 minutes
- **Ingredients:** 1 head cauliflower, grated, 1 tablespoon olive oil, 1/4 cup diced onions, 1/4 cup diced carrots, 2 cloves garlic, minced, 1/2 teaspoon turmeric, salt and pepper to taste
- **Servings:** 4
- **Cooking Method:** Sautéing
- **Procedure:** 1. Sauté onions, carrots, and garlic in olive oil. 2. Add grated cauliflower and turmeric. 3. Cook for 10 minutes. 4. Season with salt and pepper. 5. Serve warm.
- **Nutritional Values (per serving):** Calories: 70 kcal, Protein: 3g, Carbohydrates: 10g, Fat: 3g, Fiber: 3g, Sugars: 4g

Zucchini Noodle Alfredo

- **Preparation Time:** 15 minutes
- **Ingredients:** 2 large zucchinis, spiralized, 1/4 cup cashew cream, 1 garlic clove, minced, 1 tablespoon nutritional yeast, salt and pepper to taste
- **Servings:** 4
- **Cooking Method:** Sautéing
- **Procedure:** 1. Sauté garlic in a non-stick pan. 2. Add zucchini noodles, cook for 5 minutes. 3. Stir in cashew cream and nutritional yeast. 4. Season with salt and pepper. 5. Serve hot.
- **Nutritional Values (per serving):** Calories: 100 kcal, Protein: 5g, Carbohydrates: 8g, Fat: 6g, Fiber: 2g, Sugars: 3g

Sweet Potato Toasts

- **Preparation Time:** 25 minutes
- **Ingredients:** 2 large sweet potatoes, sliced, 1 tablespoon olive oil, toppings of choice (avocado, hummus, etc.)
- **Servings:** 4
- **Cooking Method:** Baking
- **Procedure:** 1. Brush sweet potato slices with olive oil. 2. Bake at 400°F for 20 minutes. 3. Add desired toppings. 4. Serve immediately.
- **Nutritional Values (per serving):** Calories: 120 kcal, Protein: 2g, Carbohydrates: 20g, Fat: 4g, Fiber: 3g, Sugars: 4g

Spaghetti Squash Primavera

- **Preparation Time:** 45 minutes
- **Ingredients:** 1 spaghetti squash, halved, 1 cup mixed vegetables (bell peppers, broccoli, etc.), 2 tablespoons olive oil, 1 teaspoon Italian seasoning, salt and pepper to taste
- **Servings:** 4
- **Cooking Method:** Baking and Sautéing
- **Procedure:** 1. Bake squash at 375°F for 40 minutes. 2. Sauté vegetables in olive oil. 3. Scrape squash into strands. 4. Combine with vegetables, season. 5. Serve warm.
- **Nutritional Values (per serving):** Calories: 150 kcal, Protein: 2g, Carbohydrates: 15g, Fat: 9g, Fiber: 4g, Sugars: 6g

Butternut Squash Gnocchi

- **Preparation Time:** 60 minutes
- **Ingredients:** 1 cup mashed butternut squash, 1/2 cup almond flour, 1/2 cup tapioca flour, salt and pepper to taste
- **Servings:** 4
- **Cooking Method:** Boiling
- **Procedure:** 1. Mix squash with flours, season. 2. Form into gnocchi shapes. 3. Boil until they float. 4. Serve with sauce of choice.
- **Nutritional Values (per serving):** Calories: 150 kcal, Protein: 3g, Carbohydrates: 25g, Fat: 5g, Fiber: 3g, Sugars: 3g

9.3. Dips and Sauces

Roasted Red Pepper Hummus

- **Preparation Time:** 15 minutes
- **Ingredients:** 1 can chickpeas, drained, 1 roasted red pepper, 2 tablespoons tahini, 1 garlic clove, juice of 1 lemon, salt to taste
- **Servings:** 4
- **Cooking Method:** Blending
- **Procedure:** 1. Combine all ingredients in a blender. 2. Blend until smooth. 3. Adjust salt to taste. 4. Serve with fresh vegetables or crackers.
- **Nutritional Values (per serving):** Calories: 120 kcal, Protein: 6g, Carbohydrates: 18g, Fat: 4g, Fiber: 5g, Sugars: 3g

Avocado Lime Dressing

- **Preparation Time:** 10 minutes
- **Ingredients:** 1 ripe avocado, juice of 2 limes, 1/4 cup olive oil, 1 garlic clove, salt and pepper to taste
- **Servings:** 4
- **Cooking Method:** Blending
- **Procedure:** 1. Scoop avocado into a blender. 2. Add lime juice, olive oil, garlic, salt, and pepper. 3. Blend until creamy. 4. Drizzle over salads or grilled meats.
- **Nutritional Values (per serving):** Calories: 150 kcal, Protein: 2g, Carbohydrates: 8g, Fat: 14g, Fiber: 4g, Sugars: 1g

Creamy Garlic Herb Dip

- **Preparation Time:** 15 minutes
- **Ingredients:** 1/2 cup Greek yogurt, 2 tablespoons chopped fresh herbs (parsley, dill), 1 garlic clove, minced, salt and pepper to taste
- **Servings:** 4
- **Cooking Method:** Mixing
- **Procedure:** 1. Combine Greek yogurt with fresh herbs and garlic. 2. Season with salt and pepper. 3. Chill for 10 minutes. 4. Serve with raw vegetables or pita chips.
- **Nutritional Values (per serving):** Calories: 35 kcal, Protein: 3g, Carbohydrates: 2g, Fat: 1g, Fiber: 0g, Sugars: 2g

Spicy Tomato Salsa

- **Preparation Time:** 20 minutes
- **Ingredients:** 3 ripe tomatoes, chopped, 1/2 onion, finely chopped, 1 jalapeño, minced, 1/4 cup cilantro, chopped, juice of 1 lime, salt to taste
- **Servings:** 4
- **Cooking Method:** Mixing
- **Procedure:** 1. Mix tomatoes, onion, jalapeño, and cilantro in a bowl. 2. Squeeze in lime juice and add salt. 3. Let it sit for 15 minutes. 4. Serve with tortilla chips or as a topping.
- **Nutritional Values (per serving):** Calories: 25 kcal, Protein: 1g, Carbohydrates: 5g, Fat: 0g, Fiber: 1g, Sugars: 3g

Cucumber Yogurt Sauce (Tzatziki)

- **Preparation Time:** 15 minutes
- **Ingredients:** 1 cup Greek yogurt, 1 cucumber, grated and drained, 2 garlic cloves, minced, 1 tablespoon olive oil, 1 tablespoon dill, salt to taste
- **Servings:** 4
- **Cooking Method:** Mixing

- **Procedure:** 1. Combine yogurt with cucumber, garlic, olive oil, and dill. 2. Season with salt. 3. Refrigerate for 1 hour. 4. Serve as a dip or sauce with grilled meats or vegetables.
- **Nutritional Values (per serving):** Calories: 70 kcal, Protein: 4g, Carbohydrates: 5g, Fat: 4g, Fiber: 0g, Sugars: 4g

Chapter 10: Delicious Desserts

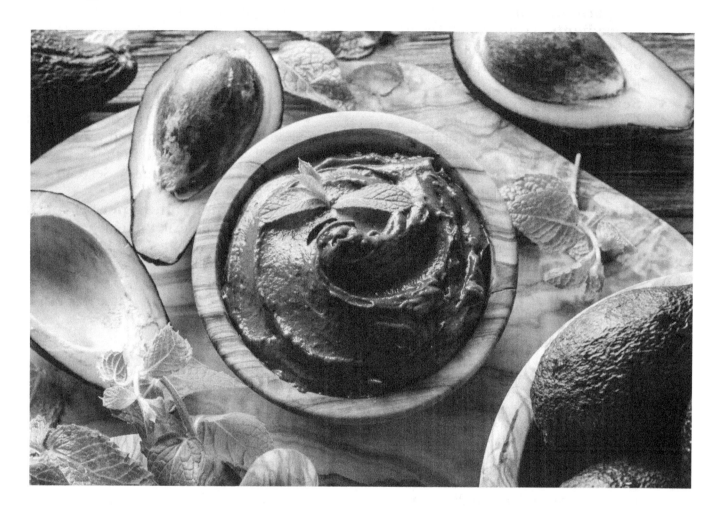

10.1. Guilt-Free Sweet Treats

Almond and Date Truffles

- **Preparation Time:** 20 minutes
- **Ingredients:** 1 cup almonds, 1 cup dates (pitted), 2 tablespoons cocoa powder, 1 teaspoon vanilla extract, pinch of salt
- **Servings:** 12 truffles
- **Cooking Method:** Blending and Rolling

- **Procedure:** 1. Pulse almonds in a food processor until finely ground. 2. Add dates, cocoa powder, vanilla, and salt, blending until sticky. 3. Roll mixture into small balls. 4. Refrigerate for 1 hour before serving.
- **Nutritional Values (per serving):** Calories: 120 kcal, Protein: 3g, Carbohydrates: 18g, Fat: 5g, Fiber: 3g, Sugars: 13g

Coconut Yogurt Parfait

- **Preparation Time:** 10 minutes
- **Ingredients:** 1 cup coconut yogurt, 1/2 cup mixed berries, 1/4 cup granola (gluten-free), 1 tablespoon honey
- **Servings:** 2
- **Cooking Method:** Layering
- **Procedure:** 1. Spoon half of the yogurt into two glasses. 2. Add a layer of berries and granola. 3. Top with remaining yogurt and drizzle with honey.
- **Nutritional Values (per serving):** Calories: 190 kcal, Protein: 6g, Carbohydrates: 28g, Fat: 7g, Fiber: 2g, Sugars: 20g

Baked Apple Chips

- **Preparation Time:** 45 minutes (including baking time)
- **Ingredients:** 2 apples, thinly sliced, 1 teaspoon cinnamon
- **Servings:** 4
- **Cooking Method:** Baking
- **Procedure:** 1. Preheat oven to 200°F (93°C). 2. Arrange apple slices on a baking sheet. 3. Sprinkle with cinnamon. 4. Bake for 40 minutes, flipping halfway.
- **Nutritional Values (per serving):** Calories: 50 kcal, Protein: 0g, Carbohydrates: 13g, Fat: 0g, Fiber: 2g, Sugars: 10g

Chocolate Avocado Mousse

- **Preparation Time:** 15 minutes
- **Ingredients:** 2 ripe avocados, 1/4 cup cocoa powder, 1/4 cup maple syrup, 1/2 teaspoon vanilla extract
- **Servings:** 4
- **Cooking Method:** Blending
- **Procedure:** 1. Blend avocados, cocoa powder, maple syrup, and vanilla until smooth. 2. Chill in the refrigerator for 1 hour. 3. Serve in small cups.
- **Nutritional Values (per serving):** Calories: 220 kcal, Protein: 3g, Carbohydrates: 27g, Fat: 12g, Fiber: 7g, Sugars: 17g

Frozen Banana Bites

- **Preparation Time:** 1 hour 30 minutes (including freezing time)
- **Ingredients:** 2 bananas, 1/4 cup dark chocolate chips, 1/4 cup peanut butter
- **Servings:** 6 bites
- **Cooking Method:** Freezing
- **Procedure:** 1. Slice bananas and sandwich with peanut butter. 2. Freeze for 1 hour. 3. Melt chocolate and dip banana bites. 4. Freeze again for 30 minutes.
- **Nutritional Values (per serving):** Calories: 150 kcal, Protein: 2g, Carbohydrates: 18g, Fat: 8g, Fiber: 2g, Sugars: 12g

10.2. Baking with Low-Fodmap Flours

Quinoa Flour Banana Bread

- **Preparation Time:** 60 minutes
- **Ingredients:** 2 ripe bananas, 1 1/2 cups quinoa flour, 1/4 cup maple syrup, 1/2 cup unsweetened almond milk, 1 tsp baking powder, 1/2 tsp cinnamon, pinch of salt
- **Servings:** 10 slices
- **Cooking Method:** Baking
- **Procedure:** 1. Preheat oven to 350°F (175°C). 2. Mash bananas and mix with maple syrup and almond milk. 3. Combine quinoa flour, baking powder, cinnamon, and salt. 4. Blend wet and dry ingredients. 5. Pour into a greased loaf pan. 6. Bake for 45 minutes.
- **Nutritional Values (per serving):** Calories: 120 kcal, Protein: 3g, Carbohydrates: 25g, Fat: 1g, Fiber: 2g, Sugars: 10g

Almond Flour Blueberry Muffins

- **Preparation Time:** 35 minutes
- **Ingredients:** 2 cups almond flour, 1/2 cup fresh blueberries, 2 eggs, 1/4 cup honey, 1 tsp vanilla extract, 1/2 tsp baking soda, pinch of salt
- **Servings:** 12 muffins
- **Cooking Method:** Baking
- **Procedure:** 1. Preheat oven to 350°F (175°C). 2. Whisk together eggs, honey, and vanilla. 3. Mix almond flour, baking soda, and salt. 4. Fold in blueberries. 5. Spoon batter into muffin tins. 6. Bake for 20 minutes.
- **Nutritional Values (per serving):** Calories: 150 kcal, Protein: 5g, Carbohydrates: 10g, Fat: 11g, Fiber: 3g, Sugars: 6g

Coconut Flour Pancakes

- **Preparation Time:** 20 minutes
- **Ingredients:** 1/2 cup coconut flour, 4 eggs, 1/2 cup coconut milk, 1 tbsp coconut oil, 2 tbsp honey, 1/2 tsp baking powder
- **Servings:** 2-3
- **Cooking Method:** Frying
- **Procedure:** 1. Whisk together eggs, coconut milk, and honey. 2. Stir in coconut flour and baking powder. 3. Heat coconut oil on a skillet. 4. Pour batter to form pancakes. 5. Cook each side for 3 minutes.
- **Nutritional Values (per serving):** Calories: 200 kcal, Protein: 6g, Carbohydrates: 18g, Fat: 12g, Fiber: 5g, Sugars: 8g

Oat Flour Apple Crisp

- **Preparation Time:** 50 minutes
- **Ingredients:** 3 apples, sliced, 1 cup oat flour, 1/2 cup brown sugar, 1/2 cup butter, 1 tsp cinnamon
- **Servings:** 6
- **Cooking Method:** Baking
- **Procedure:** 1. Preheat oven to 375°F (190°C). 2. Layer apple slices in a baking dish. 3. Mix oat flour, brown sugar, and cinnamon. 4. Cut in butter until crumbly. 5. Sprinkle over apples. 6. Bake for 30 minutes.
- **Nutritional Values (per serving):** Calories: 300 kcal, Protein: 4g, Carbohydrates: 40g, Fat: 15g, Fiber: 4g, Sugars: 25g

Rice Flour Chocolate Chip Cookies

- **Preparation Time:** 25 minutes
- **Ingredients:** 1 1/2 cups rice flour, 1/2 cup chocolate chips, 1/2 cup brown sugar, 1/4 cup butter, 1 egg, 1 tsp vanilla extract, 1/2 tsp baking soda, pinch of salt
- **Servings:** 15 cookies
- **Cooking Method:** Baking
- **Procedure:** 1. Preheat oven to 350°F (175°C). 2. Cream butter and sugar. 3. Add egg and vanilla. 4. Stir in rice flour, baking soda, and salt. 5. Mix in chocolate chips. 6. Drop spoonfuls onto baking sheet. 7. Bake for 10 minutes.
- **Nutritional Values (per serving):** Calories: 140 kcal, Protein: 2g, Carbohydrates: 20g, Fat: 6g, Fiber: 1g, Sugars: 12g

10.3. Celebratory Desserts

Raspberry Almond Tart

- **Preparation Time:** 45 minutes
- **Ingredients:** 1 cup almond flour, 1/2 cup coconut oil, 1/4 cup honey, 2 cups fresh raspberries, 1 tsp vanilla extract, pinch of salt
- **Servings:** 8
- **Cooking Method:** Baking
- **Procedure:** 1. Preheat oven to 350°F (175°C). 2. Mix almond flour, coconut oil, honey, and salt for the crust. 3. Press into a tart pan. 4. Bake for 15 minutes. 5. Arrange raspberries on the crust. 6. Chill before serving.
- **Nutritional Values (per serving):** Calories: 220 kcal, Protein: 4g, Carbohydrates: 18g, Fat: 16g, Fiber: 4g, Sugars: 10g

Chocolate Avocado Mousse

- **Preparation Time:** 15 minutes
- **Ingredients:** 2 ripe avocados, 1/4 cup cocoa powder, 1/4 cup maple syrup, 1 tsp vanilla extract, pinch of salt
- **Servings:** 4
- **Cooking Method:** Blending
- **Procedure:** 1. Blend avocados, cocoa powder, maple syrup, vanilla, and salt until smooth. 2. Chill for 1 hour. 3. Serve garnished with fruit or nuts.
- **Nutritional Values (per serving):** Calories: 230 kcal, Protein: 3g, Carbohydrates: 20g, Fat: 15g, Fiber: 7g, Sugars: 10g

Lemon Coconut Cake

- **Preparation Time:** 60 minutes
- **Ingredients:** 1 1/2 cups coconut flour, 1/2 cup honey, 4 eggs, 1/2 cup coconut oil, 1 lemon (juice and zest), 1 tsp baking powder
- **Servings:** 8
- **Cooking Method:** Baking
- **Procedure:** 1. Preheat oven to 350°F (175°C). 2. Whisk eggs, honey, lemon juice, and zest. 3. Mix in coconut flour and baking powder. 4. Bake in a greased pan for 30 minutes. 5. Cool before serving.
- **Nutritional Values (per serving):** Calories: 280 kcal, Protein: 6g, Carbohydrates: 25g, Fat: 18g, Fiber: 5g, Sugars: 15g

Flourless Chocolate Cake

- **Preparation Time:** 50 minutes
- **Ingredients:** 1 cup dark chocolate, 3/4 cup butter, 1/2 cup sugar, 4 eggs, 1 tsp vanilla extract
- **Servings:** 8
- **Cooking Method:** Baking
- **Procedure:** 1. Melt chocolate and butter together. 2. Mix in sugar, eggs, and vanilla. 3. Pour into a greased pan. 4. Bake at 325°F (160°C) for 25 minutes. 5. Cool before serving.
- **Nutritional Values (per serving):** Calories: 330 kcal, Protein: 4g, Carbohydrates: 25g, Fat: 25g, Fiber: 2g, Sugars: 20g

Strawberry Cashew Cheesecake

- **Preparation Time:** 4 hours (includes chilling time)
- **Ingredients:** 2 cups cashews (soaked), 1 cup strawberries, 1/2 cup coconut oil, 1/4 cup maple syrup, 1 lemon (juice and zest), crust: 1 cup dates, 1 cup almonds
- **Servings:** 10
- **Cooking Method:** Freezing
- **Procedure:** 1. Blend dates and almonds for crust, press into a pan. 2. Blend cashews, strawberries, coconut oil, maple syrup, lemon juice, and zest. 3. Pour over crust. 4. Freeze for 3 hours. 5. Serve chilled.
- **Nutritional Values (per serving):** Calories: 350 kcal, Protein: 6g, Carbohydrates: 30g, Fat: 24g, Fiber: 4g, Sugars: 18g

Chapter 11: Refreshing Beverages

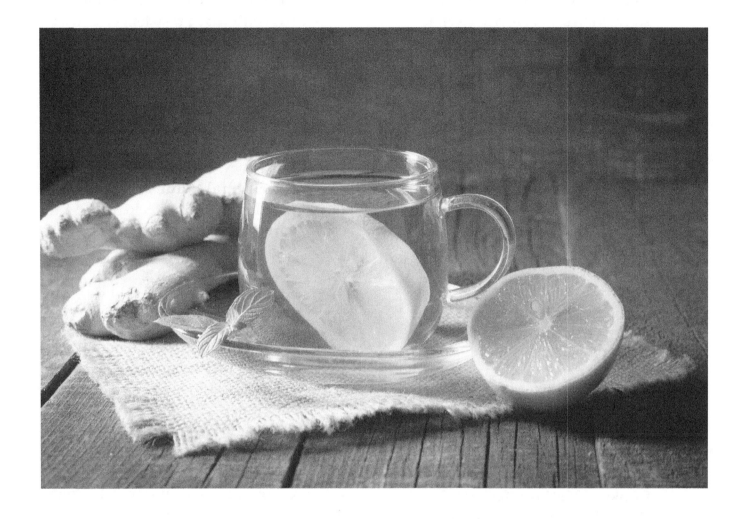

11.1. Soothing Drinks and Teas

- **Preparation Time:** 15 minutes
- **Ingredients:** 1 tbsp dried chamomile flowers, 1-inch fresh ginger root, 1 tsp honey, 2 cups water
- **Servings:** 2
- **Cooking Method:** Simmering
- **Procedure:** 1. Peel and slice ginger. 2. Boil water, add ginger and chamomile. 3. Simmer for 10 minutes. 4. Strain, add honey, and serve.

- **Nutritional Values (per serving):** Calories: 20 kcal, Protein: 0g, Carbohydrates: 5g, Fat: 0g, Fiber: 0g, Sugars: 4g

Lavender Lemon Balm Tea

- **Preparation Time:** 10 minutes
- **Ingredients:** 1 tsp dried lavender flowers, 1 tsp dried lemon balm, 2 cups boiling water
- **Servings:** 2
- **Cooking Method:** Infusing
- **Procedure:** 1. Place lavender and lemon balm in a teapot. 2. Add boiling water. 3. Steep for 5 minutes. 4. Strain and serve.
- **Nutritional Values (per serving):** Calories: 0 kcal, Protein: 0g, Carbohydrates: 0g, Fat: 0g, Fiber: 0g, Sugars: 0g

Peppermint and Licorice Root Tea

- **Preparation Time:** 15 minutes
- **Ingredients:** 1 tbsp dried peppermint leaves, 1 tsp licorice root, 2 cups water
- **Servings:** 2
- **Cooking Method:** Boiling
- **Procedure:** 1. Boil water, add peppermint and licorice root. 2. Simmer for 10 minutes. 3. Strain and serve warm.
- **Nutritional Values (per serving):** Calories: 0 kcal, Protein: 0g, Carbohydrates: 0g, Fat: 0g, Fiber: 0g, Sugars: 0g

Fennel and Honey Tea

- **Preparation Time:** 10 minutes
- **Ingredients:** 1 tbsp fennel seeds, 2 cups water, 1 tbsp honey
- **Servings:** 2
- **Cooking Method:** Simmering
- **Procedure:** 1. Crush fennel seeds slightly. 2. Boil water, add fennel seeds. 3. Simmer for 5 minutes. 4. Add honey, strain, and serve.
- **Nutritional Values (per serving):** Calories: 35 kcal, Protein: 0g, Carbohydrates: 9g, Fat: 0g, Fiber: 0g, Sugars: 8g

Turmeric and Ginger Tea

- **Preparation Time:** 20 minutes
- **Ingredients:** 1 tsp turmeric powder, 1-inch ginger root, 1 tsp lemon juice, 2 cups water, 1 tsp honey
- **Servings:** 2
- **Cooking Method:** Boiling
- **Procedure:** 1. Peel and slice ginger. 2. Boil water with ginger and turmeric for 15 minutes. 3. Add lemon juice. 4. Strain, add honey, and serve.
- **Nutritional Values (per serving):** Calories: 20 kcal, Protein: 0g, Carbohydrates: 5g, Fat: 0g, Fiber: 0g, Sugars: 4g

11.2. Healthy Smoothies and Shakes

Blueberry Spinach Smoothie

- **Preparation Time:** 10 minutes
- **Ingredients:** 1 cup fresh blueberries, 1 cup spinach leaves, 1 banana, 1/2 cup Greek yogurt, 1 cup almond milk, 1 tbsp chia seeds
- **Servings:** 2
- **Cooking Method:** Blending
- **Procedure:** 1. Combine all ingredients in a blender. 2. Blend until smooth. 3. Serve chilled.
- **Nutritional Values (per serving):** Calories: 180 kcal, Protein: 6g, Carbohydrates: 28g, Fat: 5g, Fiber: 4g, Sugars: 15g

Carrot Ginger Smoothie

- **Preparation Time:** 10 minutes
- **Ingredients:** 2 medium carrots, peeled and chopped, 1/2-inch ginger root, 1 apple, 1 cup water, 1 tbsp lemon juice, 1 tsp honey
- **Servings:** 2
- **Cooking Method:** Blending
- **Procedure:** 1. Add carrots, ginger, apple, and water to blender. 2. Blend until smooth. 3. Add lemon juice and honey, blend again.
- **Nutritional Values (per serving):** Calories: 95 kcal, Protein: 1g, Carbohydrates: 24g, Fat: 0.5g, Fiber: 5g, Sugars: 18g

Tropical Avocado Smoothie

- **Preparation Time:** 10 minutes
- **Ingredients:** 1 ripe avocado, 1/2 cup pineapple chunks, 1/2 cup mango chunks, 1 cup coconut water, 1 tbsp lime juice
- **Servings:** 2
- **Cooking Method:** Blending
- **Procedure:** 1. Scoop out avocado flesh. 2. Combine avocado, pineapple, mango, and coconut water in a blender. 3. Add lime juice, blend until creamy.
- **Nutritional Values (per serving):** Calories: 210 kcal, Protein: 3g, Carbohydrates: 30g, Fat: 10g, Fiber: 7g, Sugars: 20g

Berry Almond Milkshake

- **Preparation Time:** 10 minutes
- **Ingredients:** 1 cup mixed berries (strawberries, raspberries, blueberries), 1 cup almond milk, 1/2 cup Greek yogurt, 1 tbsp almond butter, 1 tsp vanilla extract
- **Servings:** 2
- **Cooking Method:** Blending
- **Procedure:** 1. Add all ingredients to blender. 2. Blend until smooth and creamy. 3. Serve immediately.
- **Nutritional Values (per serving):** Calories: 150 kcal, Protein: 5g, Carbohydrates: 18g, Fat: 7g, Fiber: 4g, Sugars: 12g

Cucumber Mint Smoothie

- **Preparation Time:** 10 minutes
- **Ingredients:** 1 large cucumber, peeled and sliced, 1/2 cup fresh mint leaves, 1 cup Greek yogurt, 1 tbsp honey, juice of 1 lime, 1/2 cup ice
- **Servings:** 2
- **Cooking Method:** Blending
- **Procedure:** 1. Combine cucumber, mint, yogurt, honey, lime juice, and ice in a blender. 2. Blend until smooth. 3. Serve chilled.
- **Nutritional Values (per serving):** Calories: 120 kcal, Protein: 6g, Carbohydrates: 18g, Fat: 3g, Fiber: 1g, Sugars: 15g

11.3. Low-Fodmap Cocktails and Mocktails

Ginger Peach Fizz Mocktail

- **Preparation Time:** 5 minutes
- **Ingredients:** 1 ripe peach, pitted and sliced, 1/2-inch fresh ginger, grated, 1 tbsp lemon juice, 1 tsp honey, sparkling water
- **Servings:** 2
- **Cooking Method:** Mixing
- **Procedure:** 1. Muddle peach slices and ginger in a shaker. 2. Add lemon juice and honey, shake well. 3. Strain into glasses, top with sparkling water.
- **Nutritional Values (per serving):** Calories: 50 kcal, Protein: 1g, Carbohydrates: 13g, Fat: 0g, Fiber: 1g, Sugars: 11g

Cucumber Mint Cooler

- **Preparation Time:** 10 minutes
- **Ingredients:** 1/2 cucumber, sliced, 10 mint leaves, 2 tsp lime juice, 1 tsp sugar, soda water
- **Servings:** 2
- **Cooking Method:** Mixing
- **Procedure:** 1. Combine cucumber, mint, lime juice, and sugar in a pitcher. 2. Muddle gently. 3. Add ice, top with soda water.
- **Nutritional Values (per serving):** Calories: 30 kcal, Protein: 0g, Carbohydrates: 7g, Fat: 0g, Fiber: 0.5g, Sugars: 6g

Pineapple Basil Smash

- **Preparation Time:** 5 minutes
- **Ingredients:** 1/2 cup pineapple chunks, 4 basil leaves, 1 tbsp lime juice, 1 tsp maple syrup, sparkling water
- **Servings:** 2
- **Cooking Method:** Blending
- **Procedure:** 1. Blend pineapple, basil, lime juice, and maple syrup. 2. Strain into glasses filled with ice. 3. Top with sparkling water.
- **Nutritional Values (per serving):** Calories: 60 kcal, Protein: 0.5g, Carbohydrates: 15g, Fat: 0g, Fiber: 1g, Sugars: 12g

Strawberry Lavender Lemonade

- **Preparation Time:** 15 minutes
- **Ingredients:** 1 cup strawberries, hulled, 1 tsp dried lavender, 2 tbsp lemon juice, 2 tsp sugar, water
- **Servings:** 2
- **Cooking Method:** Simmering and Mixing
- **Procedure:** 1. Simmer lavender in 1 cup water, strain. 2. Blend strawberries, lemon juice, sugar, lavender water. 3. Serve over ice.
- **Nutritional Values (per serving):** Calories: 80 kcal, Protein: 1g, Carbohydrates: 20g, Fat: 0.5g, Fiber: 2g, Sugars: 17g

Rosemary Grapefruit Spritzer

- **Preparation Time:** 10 minutes
- **Ingredients:** 1 grapefruit, juiced, 1 sprig rosemary, 1 tsp honey, sparkling water
- **Servings:** 2
- **Cooking Method:** Mixing
- **Procedure:** 1. Muddle rosemary and honey in a glass. 2. Add grapefruit juice, stir well. 3. Top with sparkling water, ice.
- **Nutritional Values (per serving):** Calories: 70 kcal, Protein: 1g, Carbohydrates: 18g, Fat: 0g, Fiber: 1g, Sugars: 16g

Chapter 12: 60-Day Meal Plan

12.1. Week-by-Week Meal Planning

As we turn the pages to Chapter 12, "60-Day Meal Plan," we embark on a pivotal phase of your Low-Fodmap journey. This chapter is designed to provide a structured, practical guide to integrating the Low-Fodmap diet into your daily life over a two-month period. It serves as a comprehensive blueprint, offering week-by-week meal planning, detailed shopping lists, preparation tips, and flexible strategies to adapt the plan to your individual needs and preferences. This introduction aims to set the stage for this crucial part of your journey, ensuring you have a clear roadmap to navigate the Low-Fodmap diet successfully.

Week-by-Week Meal Planning: A Structured Approach to Dietary Management

The cornerstone of this chapter is the week-by-week meal planning guide. This section is meticulously crafted to ease you into the Low-Fodmap diet, reducing the overwhelming task of meal planning into manageable weekly segments. Each week introduces new recipes and ideas, gradually building a diverse and satisfying dietary routine. This phased approach not only helps in slowly adapting your gut to the diet but also assists in identifying potential trigger foods as you reintroduce them.

The meal plans are designed with variety and balance in mind, ensuring that each week is not only nutritionally complete but also exciting and flavorful. This approach fosters a positive relationship with food, turning the dietary restrictions of the Low-Fodmap diet into an opportunity to explore new cuisines and flavors.

Shopping Lists and Prep Tips: Streamlining Your Dietary Transition

To complement the meal plans, this chapter provides detailed shopping lists. These lists are tailored to each week's menu, ensuring you have all the necessary ingredients on hand.

This meticulous planning aims to streamline your grocery shopping experience, making it more efficient and less stressful.

In addition to the shopping lists, you will find preparation tips and tricks. These tips are designed to make meal preparation easier and more time-efficient. Whether it's advice on batch cooking or tips on storing prepared meals, this section is packed with practical solutions to common kitchen challenges. These strategies not only save time but also help in maintaining the freshness and nutritional value of your meals.

Adapting the Plan to Your Needs: Personalization is Key

Recognizing that each individual's journey with IBS and digestive disorders is unique, this chapter emphasizes the importance of personalizing the meal plan. Adaptation strategies are provided to tailor the plan according to your specific dietary requirements, preferences, and lifestyle.

This section guides you on how to tweak recipes, substitute ingredients, and adjust meal portions to suit your needs. It also addresses common challenges such as dining out, managing busy schedules, and catering to family members not on the diet. The goal is to provide you with the flexibility to make the Low-Fodmap diet a sustainable and enjoyable part of your life.

A Journey of Empowerment and Self-Discovery

This 60-day meal plan is more than just a dietary regimen; it's a journey of empowerment and self-discovery. It equips you with the knowledge and skills to take control of your diet and, by extension, your symptoms. It encourages you to listen to your body, understand its responses to different foods, and make informed choices about what you eat.

As we move forward with this chapter, remember that the journey with the Low-Fodmap diet is a continuous learning process. There will be successes and setbacks, but each experience brings valuable insights. This 60-day plan is not just a temporary diet; it's a stepping stone towards a longer journey of health and well-being. It's about building a foundation that you can rely on as you continue to navigate the complexities of digestive health.

Chapter 12 stands as a vital component of your Low-Fodmap journey. It provides a structured yet flexible framework to integrate the diet into your life. As you delve into this chapter, approach it with an open mind, a willingness to experiment, and a commitment to your health. This 60-day meal plan is your roadmap to a life of fewer symptoms, greater comfort, and enhanced well-being.

Week 1

Day/Week	Breakfast	Lunch	Dinner	Afternoon Snack	Dessert
Monday	Ginger Peach Fizz Mocktail	Cucumber Mint Cooler	Pineapple Basil Smash	Strawberry Lavender Lemonade	Rosemary Grapefruit Spritzer
Tuesday	Strawberry Lavender Lemonade	Rosemary Grapefruit Spritzer	Ginger Peach Fizz Mocktail	Cucumber Mint Cooler	Pineapple Basil Smash
Wednesday	Pineapple Basil Smash	Strawberry Lavender Lemonade	Cucumber Mint Cooler	Rosemary Grapefruit Spritzer	Ginger Peach Fizz Mocktail
Thursday	Cucumber Mint Cooler	Pineapple Basil Smash	Rosemary Grapefruit Spritzer	Ginger Peach Fizz Mocktail	Strawberry Lavender Lemonade
Friday	Rosemary Grapefruit Spritzer	Ginger Peach Fizz Mocktail	Strawberry Lavender Lemonade	Pineapple Basil Smash	Cucumber Mint Cooler
Saturday	Strawberry Lavender Lemonade	Cucumber Mint Cooler	Pineapple Basil Smash	Ginger Peach Fizz Mocktail	Rosemary Grapefruit Spritzer
Sunday	Pineapple Basil Smash	Rosemary Grapefruit Spritzer	Ginger Peach Fizz Mocktail	Strawberry Lavender Lemonade	Cucumber Mint Cooler

Week 2

Day	Breakfast	Lunch	Dinner	Snack	Dessert
Monday	Quick Oatmeal	Quinoa Salad	Baked Salmon	Rice Cakes	Berry Sorbet
Tuesday	Smoothie Bowl	Veggie Wrap	Grilled Chicken	Mixed Nuts	Fruit Salad
Wednesday	Scrambled Eggs	Lentil Soup	Tofu Stir-Fry	Carrot Sticks	Chia Pudding
Thursday	Banana Pancakes	Chicken Salad	Beef Stew	Greek Yogurt	Almond Cookies
Friday	Granola and Yogurt	Sushi Rolls	Turkey Meatballs	Fruit Slices	Rice Pudding
Saturday	Omelette	Tuna Sandwich	Shrimp Pasta	Hummus & Veggies	Chocolate Mousse
Sunday	French Toast	Caesar Salad	Pizza with GF Base	Popcorn	Panna Cotta

Week 3

Day	Breakfast	Lunch	Dinner	Snack	Dessert
Monday	Fruit Salad	Veggie Burger	Stir-Fried Veggies	GF Crackers	Lemon Tart
Tuesday	Porridge	Greek Salad	Seafood Paella	Trail Mix	Apple Crisp
Wednesday	Muffins	Gazpacho	Veggie Curry	Cottage Cheese	Brownies
Thursday	Avocado Toast	Minestrone Soup	Chicken Kebabs	Edamame	Cheesecake
Friday	Smoothie	Caprese Salad	Lasagna (GF)	Rice Cakes	Fruit Compote
Saturday	Pancakes (GF)	Quiche (GF)	BBQ Ribs	Olives	Ice Cream (LF)
Sunday	Eggs Benedict (GF)	Caesar Wrap (GF)	Tofu & Veggies	Popcorn	Parfait

Week 4

Day	Breakfast	Lunch	Dinner	Snack	Dessert
Monday	Scrambled Tofu	Broccoli Salad	Lamb Chops	Pretzels (GF)	Sorbet
Tuesday	Cereal (GF)	Soba Noodle Salad	Stuffed Peppers	Fruit & Nut Mix	Rice Pudding
Wednesday	Chia Seed Pudding	Lentil Salad	Fish Tacos (GF)	Veggie Sticks	Custard
Thursday	Frittata	Veggie Soup	Chicken Stir-Fry	Yogurt (LF)	Pavlova
Friday	Granola (GF)	Pesto Pasta (GF)	Beef Stir-Fry	Apple Slices	Chocolate Cake
Saturday	Waffles (GF)	BLT Sandwich (GF)	Paella (GF)	Cheese Cubes	Popsicles
Sunday	Bagels (GF)	Chicken Caesar	Ratatouille	Trail Mix	Fruit Tarts

Week 5

Day	Breakfast	Lunch	Dinner	Snack	Dessert
Monday	Oats (GF)	Tomato Soup	Quiche (GF)	GF Crackers	Muffins (GF)
Tuesday	Smoothie (LF)	Taco Salad	Baked Cod	Veggie Chips	Gelato (LF)

Day	Breakfast	Lunch	Dinner	Snack	Dessert
Wednesday	Fruit Parfait	Tuna Salad	Veggie Lasagna	Dried Fruit	Compote
Thursday	Bagel with PB	Falafel Wrap	Grilled Steak	Nuts & Seeds	Cobbler (GF)
Friday	Breakfast Burrito	Spinach Salad	Chicken Parmesan	Popcorn	Ice Cream (LF)
Saturday	Omelette (GF)	Veggie Pizza (GF)	Thai Curry	Pretzels (GF)	Panna Cotta (LF)
Sunday	Pancakes (GF)	Shrimp Salad	Roast Chicken	Rice Cakes	Brownies (GF)

Week 6

Day	Breakfast	Lunch	Dinner	Snack	Dessert
Monday	Yogurt Bowl	Egg Salad	Spaghetti (GF)	GF Biscuits	Sorbet
Tuesday	Muesli (GF)	Gazpacho	Meatloaf (GF)	Kale Chips	Cupcakes (GF)
Wednesday	Toast (GF)	Quinoa Bowl	Veggie Burger (GF)	Hummus & Veggies	Mousse (LF)
Thursday	Smoothie Bowl (LF)	Veggie Sushi	Lamb Stew	Granola Bar (GF)	Custard (LF)
Friday	Avocado Toast (GF)	Greek Salad	Veggie Tacos	Trail Mix	Cookies (GF)
Saturday	Waffles (GF)	Soup & Salad	BBQ Chicken	Fruit Salad	Popsicles (LF)
Sunday	French Toast (GF)	Turkey Sandwich	Grilled Shrimp	Olives	Pudding (LF)

Week 7

Day	Breakfast	Lunch	Dinner	Snack	Dessert
Monday	Porridge (GF)	BLT (GF)	Chicken Marsala	Veggie & Dip	Fruit Tart (GF)
Tuesday	Oatmeal (GF)	Veggie Wrap (GF)	Beef Tacos	Rice Cakes	Cheesecake (LF)
Wednesday	Eggs & Toast (GF)	Caesar Salad	Roasted Veggies	Cheese & Crackers	Gelato (LF)

Day	Breakfast	Lunch	Dinner	Snack	Dessert
Thursday	Pancakes (GF)	Tomato Basil Soup	Pork Chops	Mixed Nuts	Brownies (GF)
Friday	Muffins (GF)	Avocado Salad	Seafood Pasta	Popcorn	Ice Cream (LF)
Saturday	French Toast (GF)	Chicken Salad	Veggie Stir Fry	Yogurt (LF)	Panna Cotta (LF)
Sunday	Granola & Yogurt	Tuna Sandwich	Pizza (GF)	Hummus & Veggies	Sorbet

Week 8

Day	Breakfast	Lunch	Dinner	Snack	Dessert
Monday	Scrambled Eggs (GF)	Quinoa & Veggies	Turkey Burgers	Fruit Slices	Mousse (LF)
Tuesday	Banana Bread (GF)	Greek Salad	Lamb Chops	Veggie Chips	Cobbler (GF)
Wednesday	Oatmeal (GF)	Pasta Salad (GF)	Grilled Fish	Trail Mix	Cupcakes (GF)
Thursday	Quiche (GF)	Lentil Soup	Beef Stir-Fry	Pretzels (GF)	Ice Cream (LF)
Friday	Smoothie (LF)	Sushi (GF)	Veggie Pizza (GF)	Granola Bar (GF)	Pudding (LF)
Saturday	Pancakes (GF)	Caesar Salad	Chicken Tacos	Rice Cakes	Cheesecake (LF)
Sunday	Muffins (GF)	Veggie Burger	Spaghetti (GF)	Fruit & Nut Mix	Sorbet

1. **GF** - Gluten-Free: Refers to foods that do not contain gluten, a protein found in wheat, barley, rye, and triticale. Gluten-free diets are essential for individuals with celiac disease or gluten intolerance.

2. **LF** - Low-Fodmap: Pertains to a diet that is low in "Fermentable Oligo-, Di-, Mono-saccharides And Polyols." These are short-chain carbohydrates that are poorly absorbed in the small intestine and can cause digestive discomfort in some people.

These acronyms are used to quickly indicate the dietary nature of each meal or ingredient, ensuring that they adhere to the specific requirements of a low-Fodmap and/or gluten-free diet.

12.2. Shopping Lists and Prep Tips

For individuals embarking on the Low-Fodmap journey, especially men between 30 and 50 years old aiming to alleviate digestive issues while balancing a busy lifestyle, effective planning is crucial. This chapter provides comprehensive shopping lists derived from the recipes in this cookbook, ensuring you have all the necessary ingredients for a smooth and successful dietary transition.

Essential Shopping List

Based on the diverse range of recipes provided in the previous chapters, your shopping list will include a variety of fresh produce, lean proteins, Low-Fodmap grains, and dairy substitutes. Here's a comprehensive list to get you started:

Fresh Produce:
- Green beans
- Carrots
- Bell peppers (red, green, yellow)
- Eggplant
- Zucchini
- Tomatoes
- Spinach
- Kale
- Lettuce
- Cucumbers
- Oranges
- Strawberries
- Blueberries
- Lemons
- Limes

Lean Proteins:
- Chicken breast
- Turkey

- Lean beef
- Tofu
- Tempeh
- Eggs

Low-Fodmap Grains:

- Quinoa
- Brown rice
- Oats
- Sourdough bread (spelt-based)

Dairy and Dairy Substitutes:

- Lactose-free milk
- Almond milk
- Coconut milk
- Lactose-free yogurt
- Hard cheeses (like Cheddar, Swiss)

Pantry Staples:

- Olive oil
- Garlic-infused oil
- Gluten-free pasta
- Canned tomatoes (no added sugar)
- Low-Fodmap chicken or vegetable broth
- Almond flour
- Coconut flour
- Maple syrup
- Dark chocolate (minimum 70% cocoa)

Herbs and Spices:

- Basil
- Parsley
- Cilantro

- Thyme
- Rosemary
- Chives
- Salt
- Pepper
- Paprika
- Cumin
- Turmeric

Meal Prep Tips for Success

With your kitchen stocked, dedicate a few hours each week for meal prep. Here are some tips to make this process more efficient:

1. **Batch Cooking:** Cook grains like quinoa or rice in bulk. They can be refrigerated and used as a base for various meals throughout the week.
2. **Protein Preparation:** Grill or bake lean proteins like chicken or tofu. These can be added to salads, soups, or served as main courses.
3. **Vegetable Prep:** Wash, chop, and store vegetables. Having these ready to go makes it easier to throw together a quick stir-fry or salad.
4. **Sauce and Dressing Prep:** Prepare Low-Fodmap dressings or sauces in advance. Store these in the refrigerator to add flavor to meals.
5. **Snack Preparation:** Portion out snacks like nuts or cut fruits and vegetables. Having these ready will prevent reaching for high-Fodmap options.

Adapting Your Shopping List

As you progress with your Low-Fodmap diet, you may find certain foods that you tolerate well and others that you don't. Adapt your shopping list accordingly. This personalized approach ensures that your diet caters to your specific digestive needs while also fitting into your lifestyle.

By preparing a thought-out shopping list and dedicating time to meal prep, you can seamlessly integrate the Low-Fodmap diet into your busy schedule. This approach not only helps in managing digestive issues but also ensures a nutritious and enjoyable diet. Remember, the goal is long-term health and well-being, and with these tips, you are well on your way to achieving it.

12.3. Adapting the Plan to Your Needs

Customizing Your Low-Fodmap Diet

Embarking on the Low-Fodmap journey is not a one-size-fits-all approach. Each individual's body reacts differently to various foods, and what works for one may not work for another. In this section, we delve into personalizing your Low-Fodmap meal plan to cater to your unique digestive system and lifestyle needs.

Identifying Personal Triggers

The first step in customizing your diet is identifying foods that trigger your symptoms. Begin by strictly following the Low-Fodmap diet as outlined in the earlier chapters. Then, gradually reintroduce foods, one at a time, to pinpoint which ones cause discomfort. Keep a food diary to track your reactions, which will be invaluable in tailoring your diet.

Aligning with Your Lifestyle

Balancing a Low-Fodmap diet with a busy lifestyle requires thoughtful planning. If you have a hectic work schedule, consider preparing meals in advance during weekends. For those who travel frequently, researching Low-Fodmap friendly restaurants or packing suitable snacks can be a game-changer.

Flexibility and Experimentation

The beauty of the Low-Fodmap diet lies in its flexibility. There are countless substitutes for high-Fodmap ingredients that don't compromise on taste.

Experiment with almond flour instead of wheat flour, or try lactose-free dairy products. The cookbook provides numerous creative recipes using these alternatives.

Your body's response to certain foods can change over time. What may have been a trigger a month ago might not cause issues now. Regularly reassess your tolerance levels and adjust your diet accordingly. This dynamic approach ensures that your diet evolves with your body's needs.

Incorporating Mindful Eating

Mindful eating is a powerful tool in managing digestive issues. It involves eating slowly, chewing thoroughly, and being fully present during meals. This practice can enhance digestion and reduce symptoms.

Recognize the emotional aspect of eating. Food is not just about sustenance; it's also about pleasure, social connections, and traditions. Adapting your Low-Fodmap diet should not mean giving up these joys. Find ways to modify your favorite recipes to fit within the diet's parameters.

Stay informed about the latest Low-Fodmap research and recipes. The diet is continuously evolving, and new findings can offer more options and flexibility.

Support Systems

Build a support system of fellow Low-Fodmap dieters. Sharing experiences, recipes, and tips can make the journey less daunting and more enjoyable.

Professional Guidance

Consider consulting a dietitian specializing in Low-Fodmap diets. They can provide personalized advice and help you navigate complex dietary decisions.

In conclusion, adapting the Low-Fodmap meal plan to your individual needs is a journey of exploration, learning, and adjustment. It's about finding the right balance that works for your body and lifestyle. By doing so, you can enjoy a varied, nutritious diet that supports your digestive health and overall well-being. Remember, the key is flexibility, experimentation, and listening to your body – this is your personal path to digestive bliss and a happier, healthier life.

As we conclude Chapter 12, "60-Day Meal Plan," it is time to reflect on the comprehensive journey we have embarked upon, encompassing week-by-week meal planning, detailed shopping lists and preparation tips, and the crucial aspect of personalizing the plan to individual needs. This concluding section aims to reinforce the key learnings and insights, ensuring that the transition to a Low-Fodmap lifestyle is not just a temporary phase but a sustainable and enjoyable part of your ongoing journey towards better digestive health and overall well-being.

Consolidating the Week-by-Week Meal Planning Approach

Throughout the 60-day period, the structured meal planning approach has served as a guiding light, offering a balanced and varied diet that caters to the requirements of a Low-Fodmap regimen. The importance of this structure cannot be overstated – it has provided a framework to ensure nutritional adequacy, introduce culinary diversity, and prevent the monotony often associated with dietary restrictions. This methodical approach has likely introduced you to new ingredients and recipes, broadening your culinary horizons and enriching your diet beyond its initial limitations.

Reflecting on the Shopping and Preparation Journey

The shopping lists and preparation tips included in this chapter were designed to streamline the often-daunting task of grocery shopping and meal prep. They have been instrumental in making the Low-Fodmap diet accessible and manageable, even for those with the busiest of schedules. The emphasis on preparation, from batch cooking to effective storage techniques, has not only saved time but also ensured that you always have Low-Fodmap friendly meals at your disposal. This level of preparedness is key in avoiding dietary slip-ups and managing symptoms effectively.

Embracing Personalization in Your Diet

One of the most crucial aspects of this journey has been the emphasis on personalization. Adapting the meal plan to fit individual lifestyles, taste preferences, and specific dietary needs is what transforms the Low-Fodmap diet from a prescriptive set of guidelines into a liveable, flexible eating plan. This personalization is what makes the diet sustainable in the long term, allowing it to evolve as your needs and circumstances change.

The Journey Beyond 60 Days

As this 60-day plan concludes, it is important to view it not as the end, but as the beginning of a continued journey with the Low-Fodmap diet. The habits, skills, and knowledge you have acquired over these two months lay the foundation for a long-term approach to managing your digestive health.

Facing Challenges and Celebrating Successes

It is natural to encounter challenges as you continue with the Low-Fodmap diet beyond this structured plan. There may be times when you inadvertently consume high-Fodmap foods or face difficulties in maintaining the diet due to life's unpredictable nature. It is important to approach these challenges with patience and resilience, learning from each experience and using it to further fine-tune your diet.

Celebrating your successes is equally important. Whether it's noticing a reduction in symptoms, enjoying a new recipe, or successfully navigating a social dining situation, each of these successes is a testament to your commitment and adaptability.

Continued Learning and Growth

The Low-Fodmap journey is one of continual learning and growth. Staying informed about the latest research, being open to trying new Low-Fodmap foods as they become available, and continually listening to your body are key to maintaining and enhancing your diet. Engaging with the Low-Fodmap community, whether through online forums, support groups, or with healthcare professionals, can provide additional support and inspiration.

Final Thoughts

As we close this chapter, remember that the journey with the Low-Fodmap diet is deeply personal and unique to each individual. It's a journey that requires commitment, but it also offers great rewards in terms of improved health and well-being. The skills, knowledge, and habits you have developed over these 60 days are tools that you can carry forward, adapting and refining them as you continue on your path to better digestive health.

In conclusion, this 60-day meal plan is just the beginning of a lifelong journey of discovery, health, and enjoyment. It's a journey that not only promises relief from digestive discomfort but also opens the doors to a more mindful, healthful, and joyful way of living. As you move forward, do so with confidence, knowing that you are well-equipped to manage your diet and your health, now and in the future.

Chapter 13: Conclusion: Embracing Your Low-Fodmap Life

13.1. Maintaining Your Low-Fodmap Diet

Integrating the Diet into Your Everyday Routine

Embarking on the Low-Fodmap journey isn't just about changing what you eat; it's about transforming your lifestyle. For many men in their 30s to 50s, daily routines are often packed with professional commitments and personal responsibilities. Integrating a Low-Fodmap diet into this busy schedule requires more than just willpower; it demands a strategic approach to meal planning and preparation.

Start by reassessing your weekly routine. Identify times when you can shop for and prepare Low-Fodmap meals. Perhaps Sunday afternoons could be your meal prep time, ensuring you have digestively friendly meals ready for the hectic work week. Keep your kitchen stocked with Low-Fodmap staples, so you always have something safe and satisfying to eat. Investing in some quality kitchen equipment, like a slow cooker or a good blender, can also make preparing Low-Fodmap meals more efficient and enjoyable.

Adapting to Social Situations and Dining Out

One of the challenges you may face is maintaining your diet in social situations. Whether it's a business lunch, a family gathering, or dinner with friends, these scenarios can often present the most significant temptation to stray from your Low-Fodmap regimen. But, with a bit of planning and confidence, you can navigate these situations successfully.

Before attending a social event, eat a small Low-Fodmap snack to curb hunger and avoid being tempted by off-limits foods. When dining out, don't hesitate to ask the server about the ingredients in dishes and request modifications if needed. Remember, many restaurants are now more accommodating to dietary restrictions. You can also suggest restaurants you know have Low-Fodmap friendly options when planning outings with friends or colleagues.

Evolving Your Diet with Time and Experience

As you become more accustomed to the Low-Fodmap diet, you'll start to notice patterns and learn which foods you can tolerate better than others. This understanding will allow you to gradually reintroduce certain foods back into your diet while still maintaining overall digestive wellness.

Keep a food diary to track your meals and any symptoms you experience. This practice will help you identify any foods that might trigger discomfort, enabling you to fine-tune your diet to your specific needs. Additionally, don't shy away from experimenting with new recipes and food combinations. The Low-Fodmap diet doesn't have to be restrictive; it can be an exciting culinary journey full of discovery and satisfaction.

Maintaining your Low-Fodmap diet is an ongoing process of learning, adapting, and finding balance in your daily life. By embracing this diet as part of your routine, staying prepared for social situations, and evolving your dietary choices based on personal experience, you'll find that managing digestive issues becomes more effortless and more integrated into your busy lifestyle. Remember, this diet isn't just about avoiding discomfort; it's about embracing a healthier, happier you.

13.2. Building a Supportive Community

When embarking on a journey like the Low-Fodmap diet, the support of a community can be as nourishing as the diet itself. The journey, while rewarding, can sometimes feel isolating, especially when it requires significant lifestyle changes. Building a supportive community not only provides encouragement but also offers a wealth of shared knowledge and experiences.

Engage with online forums and social media groups dedicated to the Low-Fodmap lifestyle. These platforms are a treasure trove of advice, recipes, and moral support. Sharing your own experiences, challenges, and triumphs not only contributes to the collective wisdom but also reinforces your own commitment to this lifestyle change.

Creating a Low-Fodmap-Friendly Environment at Home and Work

For most men in their 30s to 50s, much of life revolves around family and work. Therefore, it's crucial to cultivate an environment both at home and in the workplace that supports your dietary needs. At home, involve your family in your Low-Fodmap journey. Educate them about the diet's benefits and involve them in meal planning and preparation. This not only eases your burden but also turns mealtime into an opportunity for bonding and learning.

In the workplace, be open about your dietary needs. You'll be surprised how accommodating colleagues can be once they understand your situation. Perhaps suggest a Low-Fodmap option for the next office lunch or initiate a health-focused discussion group. These small steps can create a more inclusive and supportive environment, making it easier for you to maintain your diet.

Expanding Your Support Beyond the Immediate Circle

The journey with the Low-Fodmap diet is not just about managing a diet; it's about embracing a healthier lifestyle. To further this goal, extend your community beyond immediate circles. Participate in local health and wellness events, or join a cooking class focused on Low-Fodmap recipes. Volunteering for health-focused charities or groups can also be incredibly rewarding.

Additionally, consider starting a local support group or a cooking club for individuals on similar dietary journeys. Such initiatives not only foster community spirit but also provide a platform for collective learning and support. It's through these broader engagements that you can advocate for more widespread awareness and acceptance of the Low-Fodmap lifestyle, making it easier for everyone who chooses this path.

In conclusion, building a supportive community is a crucial aspect of successfully embracing a Low-Fodmap life. It involves nurturing connections, creating supportive environments at home and work, and expanding your support network. By doing so, you transform your diet from a personal challenge into a shared journey, enriched with camaraderie, understanding, and mutual support. Remember, while the diet is about what you eat, its success is significantly bolstered by who surrounds you and how they support your journey towards better health and wellbeing.

13.3. Looking Ahead: Long-Term Health and Happiness

The journey through a Low-Fodmap lifestyle is not just a short-term remedy; it's a gateway to long-term health and happiness. As you move forward, the principles and habits you've cultivated will become cornerstones of a sustainable, health-conscious life. This path leads not only to reduced digestive discomfort but also to enhanced overall well-being.

The key is to see the Low-Fodmap diet not as a restrictive set of rules, but as a blueprint for a more mindful and health-focused life. Over time, you'll discover that this diet enhances your understanding of nutrition, leading to improved choices that benefit your entire body, not just your digestive system. This holistic approach is what transforms a diet into a lifestyle, one that promises lasting health benefits.

Integrating Mindfulness and Wellness Beyond Diet

Your Low-Fodmap journey has equipped you with the tools to make informed dietary choices. Now, extend these principles of mindfulness and wellness to other aspects of your life. Incorporate regular exercise, stress management techniques, and adequate sleep into your routine. These elements work synergistically with your diet to promote a healthier, more balanced life.

Exercise, in particular, plays a critical role in maintaining digestive health. Activities like walking, yoga, or swimming can significantly improve gut motility and reduce stress, a known trigger for digestive issues. Similarly, practices like meditation and deep breathing exercises can help in managing stress and improving mental health, further contributing to your digestive wellness.

Continued Learning and Adaptation

The field of nutrition and digestive health is continually evolving, and staying informed about the latest research and recommendations is vital. Keep educating yourself about the Low-Fodmap diet and its developments. Books, seminars, health blogs, and consultations with healthcare professionals can provide valuable insights into further refining your diet for optimal health.

Adaptation is also key. As your body changes and life evolves, so too might your dietary needs. Be open to tweaking your diet, trying new recipes, and incorporating new Low-Fodmap foods as they become available. Remember, the goal is not just to follow a diet but to lead a life of health and happiness.

In conclusion, as you look ahead, envision a future where the Low-Fodmap diet is more than just a way to manage digestive issues—it's a foundation for a healthier, happier life. By embracing a holistic approach that includes mindful eating, regular exercise, stress management, and continual learning, you set the stage for long-term health and well-being. This journey is not just about alleviating symptoms; it's about enriching your life in every aspect, ensuring a future full of vitality and joy.

Measurement Conversion Table

Volume Equivalents (Liquid)

US Standard	US Standard (ounces)	Metric (approximate)
2 tablespoons	1 fl. oz.	30 mL
¼ cup	2 fl. oz.	60 mL
half cup	4 fl. oz.	120 mL
1 cup	8 fl. oz.	240 mL
1 half cups	12 fl. oz.	355 mL
2 cups or 1 pint	16 fl. oz.	457 mL
4 cups or 1 quart	32 fl. oz.	1 L
1 gallon	128 fl. oz.	4 L

Volume Equivalents (Dry)

US Standard	Metric (approximate)
1/8 teaspoon	0.5 mL
¼ teaspoon	1 mL
half teaspoon	2 mL
¾ teaspoon	4 mL
1 teaspoon	5 mL
1 tablespoon	15 mL
¼ cup	59 mL
1/3 cup	79 mL
half cup	118 mL
2/3 cup	156 mL
¾ cup	177 mL
1 cup	235 mL
2 cups or 1 pint	475 mL
3 cups	700 mL
4 cups or 1 quart	1 L

Oven Temperatures

Fahrenheit (F)	Celsius (C) (approximate)
250°F	120°C
300°F	150°C
325°F	165°C
350°F	180°C
375°F	190°C
400°F	200°C
425°F	220°C
450°F	230°C

Weight Equivalents

US Standard	Metric (approximate)
1 tablespoon	15 g
half ounce	15 g
1 ounce	30 g
2 ounces	60 g
4 ounces	115 g
8 ounces	225 g
12 ounces	340 g
16 ounces or 1 pound or 1 lb	455 g